why me

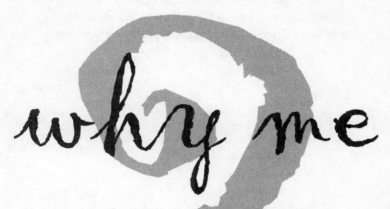

why me?

The Real-life Guide to Infertility

Loraine Brown

SIMON & SCHUSTER
AUSTRALIA

Dedication

For my mother who taught me to be a mother,
for my son who lets me practise,
and for his two special mothers, who enrich his life,
and weren't so fortunate in their quest for maternity.

WHY ME?

First published in Australasia in 1998 by
Simon & Schuster Australia
20 Barcoo Street, East Roseville NSW 2069

A Viacom Company
Sydney   New York   London   Toronto   Tokyo   Singapore

National Library of Australia
Cataloguing-in-Publication data

Brown, Loraine.
    Why me? : the real-life guide to infertility.

    Includes index.
    ISBN 0 7318 0687 5.

    1. Infertility — Popular works. 2. Infertility — Treatment
    — Popular works. 3. Infertility — Alternative treatment —
    Popular works. 4. Infertility — Psychological aspects —
    Popular works. I. Title.

616.692

Cover design: Siobhan O'Connor
Design: Anna Soo
Typeset in 10/13 pt Sabon
Printed in Australia by Australian Printing Group

Contents

Acknowledgments

Thank you to all the people who shared the intimacies of their infertility and its impact on their lives. From the far north of Queensland to the north of England, they answered my endless questions with honesty and humour, and touched me deeply.

Special thanks to Dr Stephen Steigrad, Director of the Department of Reproductive Medicine, the Royal Hospital for Women, Randwick, New South Wales, and his colleague, Eva Durna; to Leonie McMahon, Paul Entwistle, Marie Jones; to Sandra Dill from ACCESS; and to Jo Kaplan from CHILD. Thanks also to Professors Carl Wood and Robert Jansen for answering my questions.

Thanks to Robert Littell for computerising me and to Zanna Northam, from Harry M. Miller & Co. Management, whose energy was crucial in the early stages.

To my sister Carolyn, who came on the first and last interview with me and shared the journey.

And to Brian, who prompted me to write this book.

Chapter 1
My Story

I was the classic baby boomer living in the
1980s. I had everything, but nothing. I didn't have a baby.

Today as I finished this book, the residual feeling I had was one of pain from the experiences of infertility, and the experiences of those who shared their stories with me. I wonder why the sadness, as I am one of the lucky ones, with a captivating small son. I also question why, in the vivid dreams I've had during the book's gestation, it is the most painful moments I've revisited, not the joyous ones I experience every day. Perhaps it would be stating the obvious to say that having a child is worth all the pain. I asked myself if I should write a chapter on the pure joy a wanted child brings, but then I realised that for all those parents who have been to hell and back to have their children, the pleasure they now experience will in no way diminish the journey.

In my early days of wanting a child, I'd browse through books on the subject in the bookstore. If I found the author was a happy mother or father of three easily conceived children, I put the book straight down, thinking they couldn't possibly understand what I was going through. Similarly, if the author was an unsuccessful recipient of infertility treatment, I didn't want to know. I needed only good news to boost my own fragile hopes. To write about my own journey though, first I have to recall my earlier struggle with fertility.

Ten years ago, I had it all — except a baby. Not that anyone would have noticed an aching hole. I was so good at smiling through the perfume launches, advertising meetings and calming everyone else through the deadlines that not even those closest to me would have guessed. I had a job I adored — creating a wonderful, living creature called *Mode* magazine. The staff were mostly like a close group of supportive friends, united in creating a product about which we were passionate.

I had a strong partnership at home — a professional equal working in national television who was a successful writer as well. My partner loved my successes and hardly ever resented the fact that publishing took much of my time and most of my mental energy. We had a pretty inner-city stone house with a cottage annexe (my wardrobe, he called it), plus a classic whitewashed Greek island holiday home and, later, an ancient farmhouse in a hilltop village in central France.

We went to every good party in town and met the most interesting people. We travelled when I could get away. All this and a wonderfully close family with a niece and nephews to spoil and enjoy when I felt clucky.

So why did a baby seem so necessary? And why did my life seem like nothing without

1

it? I didn't ever admit it, even to my partner. He had a grown son from a previous marriage, so didn't feel great reproductive urges.

All reluctantly childless people develop a wonderful line of patter to cover up. My favourite was: 'Every time I decide it's time to have a baby, Kerry Packer gives me a new magazine to look after.'

I never really worked out why the longing for a child was so intense. It certainly wasn't the kind of trophy baby that was so popular at the time — like the latest fashion accessory. I just had a primitive, all-encompassing need to have a child, although it wasn't like that in the beginning.

My gynaecological history reads like a one-woman disaster chronicle of a baby-boomer who couldn't take the Pill — it made me depressed, it made me swollen and it made me totally disinterested in sex. I found a professor who was experimenting with the creation of low-dosage contraceptive pills, trying to tailor the hormone cocktail to suit individual patients. He was a wonderful man and his work in the 1970s may have contributed to the Pill of today. But still it didn't suit me.

Each visit I left his office with metres of cellophane strips filled with pills of different colours and instructions on which colours to take when. It was interesting, the only drawback was having to take your temperature daily and record it for medical research, noting side-effects along the way. It also brought about the first of my many temperature charts, the basal (early morning) body temperature indicating if and when ovulation occurred. This was fine for a while, but I wasn't very diligent about filling in the temperature records and the professor's partner was his ferocious (to me) wife, who clearly knew I'd made up my temperature charts. She didn't really approve of the sexual revolution or of a young woman like me wanting to stay unmarried and childless at this point.

Why is this relevant? It started off my temperature-taking — so necessary later for fertility treatment — and an awareness of my hormonal make-up.

In a settled relationship, I decided to try a diaphragm. There was a lot of anti-Pill talk which also worried me. The diaphragm took commitment and a sense of humour. My partner took great delight in hurling it around the room like a flying saucer. It worked, until the day I had only half the amount of anti-sperm cream. I took half a risk and was pregnant. I was in no way ready to become a mother, my career was too important, I felt I was too young at the age of 23.

By then, pregnancy terminations were legally possible, but only if you had a psychiatrist's report saying continuing the pregnancy was a danger to your mental health. I went along to the recommended tame psychiatrist nervously prepared to say I was contemplating suicide. Instead he asked me nice questions about my parents and family. Yes, of course I adored them and had a great relationship with them. He told me I'd failed miserably, would make a great mother, but since I wasn't ready to be one yet, he'd give me the letter. I felt tricked and humiliated. This was the time of the release of Germaine Greer's *The Female Eunuch*, so women's lib feelings were running high.

The morning of the termination, my normally loving boyfriend was suddenly really unpleasant. He took me silently to the hospital and I sat beside him filled with outrage at his behaviour. When later he came to collect me, he admitted (lovingly) that when he had been in this situation once before, he had been nice to his partner beforehand and she decided not to have the termination, so he didn't want to take that chance again!

Afterwards, my main reaction was of overwhelming relief at not feeling sick — morning sickness seemed to last all day with me, like a permanent hangover.

It was at this time that someone told me of a trendy young doctor who had a new kind of intra-uterine contraceptive device he was fitting into young women who hadn't yet had children. This was a breakthrough, as this intra-uterine device was hailed as being almost as safe as the contraceptive pill. Unfortunately, it was the now notorious Dalkon Shield, responsible for litigation all over the world by the women whose reproductive lives it destroyed.

Back then, however, it seemed like the answer to a girl's prayer. In the doctor's fashionable office, he examined me and we made arrangements for me to go into hospital and have the device fitted after a routine D&C (dilation and curettage). It was about a month after my pregnancy termination and, although my boyfriend and I had been careful, I was glad of the idea of another D&C, fear of pregnancy having become a bogeyman by then.

Stupidly, I didn't give them the urine sample they asked for, thinking that even if I was again pregnant I wouldn't be after the D&C. I remember feeling embarrassed about the whole subject of unwanted pregnancy. After the device was fitted, I waited and waited for my period to come, but knew my body was totally confused by the interventions. I was a bit surprised that my breasts were still swollen, but figured it was some kind of hormonal adjustment — after all, that's what the Pill had done to me. Finally, I went back to the doctor and he took a pregnancy test, which showed negative. He made an appointment for the following week, to investigate further.

I spent the weekend before the follow-up appointment at home with my parents in the country. Cramps and spotting started and I was relieved a period had finally come. When severe pains and serious haemorrhaging started, however, I knew it was much more. I had my sister telephone my boyfriend so that he could ring my city doctor for instructions, while she drove me to Sydney wrapped in the biggest bath towels in the house. My boyfriend was white-faced when we arrived and told me later the doctor had said I could die on the way to the city. They took me straight to the emergency room in a major women's hospital. I was sure the intra-uterine device had pierced my uterus and I wouldn't be able to have children.

A very matter-of-fact duty doctor started to examine me, with a running commentary which went something like this: 'How much blood have you lost? Five towels, you mean five sanitary towels?'

'No, bath towels,' I said.

'So, you have an IUD,' he replied.

'Yes,' I affirmed, 'a Dalkon Shield.'

'No,' he said, 'I mean an intra-uterine death, not a contraceptive device.'

'It's not possible,' I replied, 'I had a D&C and have since had a negative pregnancy test.'

'Well you have,' he told me, as he fished around. 'Look, here's a bit of placenta ...' and so the commentary went on, sensitivity not high on the agenda.

I spent the night very spaced out from lack of blood, waiting to have my own doctor come in the morning and mop up, fix the blood transfusion and explain everything. He never really did. He said I had been six weeks pregnant (dating after the intra-uterine device had been installed). However, when I was talking to the nurses, they said that I had been ten to twelve weeks pregnant, which meant that I had never had the precautionary D&C before the Dalkon Shield was fitted.

My doctor's after-care was sufficiently distracting—technically not quite breaking his Hippocratic oath—and I was too traumatised by the experience to investigate further. I was just relieved that I could still have children in the future. Although subsequent intra-uterine devices (not Dalkon Shields) actually gave me a trauma-free period from fertility to concentrate on my career, these episodes guaranteed that the whole subject of pregnancy would always carry with it some overtones of trauma.

Also, I had been born in chaos, premature and in the breech position, and my mother had had a similar bloody journey to Sydney to have me. We had both nearly died and she was told she should have no more children. So pregnancy was hardly a happy topic in my life.

When the time came for me to change my intra-uterine device, I decided I was very grown up and would change doctors. The new doctor was as chilly as the first one had been warm.

'How long have you been using an intra-uterine device?' he asked.

'Oh, almost ten years,' I replied casually.

'Oh well,' he said cheerfully, 'you probably don't need a new one now, you are probably sterile with blocked tubes.'

At this point, my attitude towards having a baby changed. It was no longer something that I could postpone indefinitely.

By this time my career was established, I was Editor of *Belle* magazine, in my early 30s and had met the man who is now my husband. He was the first man with whom I'd truly felt I could make a life and create a family. After the device was removed, I didn't do anything about contraception. I felt it was time to let fate take its course.

As my partner already had a son from a previous marriage and I'd had pregnancies, I assumed I'd be pregnant the first month. Amazingly, nothing happened. Month after month, nothing happened. At first, I thought it was because his television work took him away from home often and we were just not synchronised with my fertile times. Then I went out and bought a thermometer and made myself a chart, mindful of the instructions I'd had from the professor all those years ago — temperature first thing before putting your feet out of bed or moving.

I also bought a book on infertility, a slim volume which repeated much of the stuff I already knew — from trying *not* to get pregnant. My temperature chart looked classic, as though I was ovulating. I thought I just needed to fine-tune the timing a bit. It was amazing the number of times my partner had a 'headache' at the appropriate time. He didn't say much, knowing from the start that children were part of my life plan. As he had a son already, however, he didn't feel the need to procreate again. I still didn't discuss my non-pregnancy with him, thinking it would just happen, and he'd be pleased anyway.

By then I was in charge of four small magazines: *Belle*, *Mode*, *Mode Brides* and *Gourmet*. My staff used to call me the Managing Editor of Food, Fashion, Furniture and Fornication.

Still no pregnancy.

One false alarm and an overdue period, a scan showing a possible tubal pregnancy. Another dash to hospital for emergency surgery with my wonderful new doctor at Sydney's Royal Hospital for Women, where I was born. It wasn't a tubal pregnancy, just a late and large ovulation; I didn't lose a tube, but had fibroids removed to help later pregnancy attempts. This was followed by a fragile period recovering from surgery, but feeling glad that the two tubes were still intact.

Fibroids, a new problem I didn't know I had. I was assured, however, that a pregnancy was still possible. I did feel a gynaecological mess, but none of this stopped the production of magazines. They still dominated my life — from the hospital bed, to a light box and transparencies and layouts all over my bed at home. I put the idea of pregnancy on hold for a while to let my body recover and threw myself into re-launching *Mode* as a women's fashion newspaper, trotting out the cliches anytime anyone asked if I planned to have a family. Mostly they didn't ask, they assumed our joint careers were enough for us. My mother even gave all my doll's clothes and books to my sister's children, assuming I wasn't going to have children. I wasn't happy about that!

I didn't want to admit, even to my partner, how much I wanted a baby, so I tried to drown it all in deadlines. Magazines are greedy things, magazine people are often needy emotionally, so I was more than busy.

I made my own diagnosis, thinking the stress and travel in both our work was inhibiting things. I bullied my doctor into a prescription for Clomid (an ovulation inducing drug) — from my reading I'd worked out that this would guarantee ovulation and pinpoint the time. Then I took it during a month I was sure we'd both be in the same place at the appropriate time.

Amazingly, two weeks later, my period didn't come; a week after that, my doctor did a pregnancy test that was positive. I blissfully bought a pair of bootees, wrapped them and presented them to my partner when I got home from work. I should have known he hates surprises, even though logic would tell you that if you have unprotected intercourse with a long-term partner a child could be the outcome. He said the shattering words: 'Well, I don't want another child, so you'd better have an abortion.'

With that and a mother in hospital with breast cancer, who knows, about three days later I started to bleed. A scan delivered the message the pregnancy was not viable. There was no heartbeat. My minuscule baby was really what they call a blighted ovum. Even the words had a damning effect — blighted — barren woman — or at least that is how I felt. I also felt emptier than I'd ever felt before.

The next eighteen months were rocky ones in our relationship. We nearly didn't survive. Then we began a new phase of our lives where a child was a stated aim for both of us and I took the Clomid again. Again I was pregnant, this time with the full support of my partner. And this time an early scan revealed two foetal sacs. That day I went off to Kerry Packer's birthday lunch hugging the news of my twins to myself. We went on holiday and I carefully didn't drink alcohol or coffee, did everything I thought might help. I felt great, I didn't even feel sick. Unfortunately, I didn't realise that was *not* a good sign.

All went well until I was standing doing the dishes after a Christmas lunch I'd given for the staff. Thai chicken for twenty. I went to the loo and there was a dreaded pinkish stain on my knickers. I went straight to bed, hoping that rest would fix it. It didn't, but as my breasts were still swollen, I figured the pregnancy was still ongoing.

Back in the ultrasound unit, a place I had learned to dread. The same diagnosis: no heartbeats, no babies. Back into hospital the next day to have the dreams scraped away, the sense of loss and emptiness indescribable.

And back to the inevitable deadlines, although this time they didn't compensate. I lost my capacity to cry forever. There is rarely an adequate explanation for these pregnancies that fail to develop. The doctors tell you that statistically one in five or six pregnancies end this way, that it is nature's way of preventing damaged foetuses being born. But this is hardly satisfactory. You really want an answer, something positive that can be fixed next time.

My partner finally told me he'd had treatment to have his first child, so we decided it was time to see a fertility specialist. We both had problems and I was now thirty-seven. Time was becoming increasingly important.

Running a magazine in a competitive market is hardly the most relaxing thing to do—but it was what I did. It never occurred to me that I couldn't have this and a baby, too. One evening I went to dinner with a friend—a successful businesswoman who had also had a series of miscarriages. She had picked me up after work. I was pale and tired, having just finished an issue of the magazine. She became really angry with me and said something like, 'What right have you got to have it all—maybe you might have to give something up if you want this baby so badly.'

It was truly the first time it had occurred to me. I resolved then that if I managed to become pregnant again I would stop everything, even if it was just to make myself feel I'd done everything possible to have a baby.

The then publisher, Richard Walsh, a trained doctor, was at his best with this. He insisted I was under orders next time to stay at home and take it easy. I was far from sure there would be a next time.

We began investigations at a private clinic — starting with a sperm test and a post-coital test, dashing across Sydney with the container in a discreet brown paper bag to get to the laboratory at the prescribed time.

My partner was away when I went for the results. The doctor, with a colourful Australian turn of phrase, explained the sperm analysis thus: 'Imagine Robert De Castella (the then famous Australian marathon runner) in the centre of a group of amateur runners at the City to Surf (the annual fun run between Sydney and Bondi). Deek could run as fast as he liked, but surrounded by a mass of amateurs, he'd have trouble getting anywhere. Well, that is what the sperm are like, there are good ones there, but they have trouble getting through the others.' He told me they could separate the good ones and have them inseminated artificially into me at the clinic. If that didn't work, another option would be GIFT, where the egg and sperm are united clinically in the tube. He explained, however, that they had had a lot of multiple births the previous year with that technique. I dearly wanted one or two babies, but the thought of a litter appalled me, knowing our partnership would never survive that.

I went back to my gynaecologist and told him the news, but that I wasn't crazy about the abruptness of the doctor. He said he'd pass me over to his colleague Dr Stephen Steigrad and the Royal Hospital for Women's Fertility Clinic.

And it is them we have to thank for our son.

Ever thorough, Dr Steigrad began investigations on both of us from scratch, and yet again I had to reach for the thermometer in the mornings to do three months of temperature charts. Three months seemed an eternity, I just wanted to get started.

A laparoscopy came next to view the state of my internal organs. He did find masses of small fibroids, which made my uterus sound like a moonscape, but said they shouldn't inhibit a pregnancy.

I was a bit nonplussed when he told me in the hospital after the laparoscopy, and the head nurse must have sensed this. 'Don't worry, dear,' she said. 'He hasn't got much of a bedside manner, but if you want a baby, he's the *best*.' I felt wonderfully reassured. I was lucky. It took only four months to conceive our son. I was fortunate, too, that we lived very close to the hospital for the morning blood tests to pinpoint ovulation time and the subsequent inseminations.

In those preceding years, I had sought every kind of help — from fortune tellers to rock crystals, to vitamins and natural therapy, to privately lighting candles in churches or temples anywhere I happened to be from Notre Dame in Paris to ancient temples in Thailand. I was prepared to take help from everywhere. I also read anything I could get my hands on on the subject of fertility.

One plane trip back from Europe I happened to pick up a copy of the British edition of *Good Housekeeping* — like every magazine editor, I am a junkie for other magazines. I came across a story called 'The Fertile Mind'. And it started me thinking.

Some time earlier I had been to a general practitioner who specialised in vitamin therapy and he questioned me about my birth circumstances. When I told him it had been traumatic, he looked at me piercingly and said that this may have affected me — 'You were there, you know'. He gave me a kind of self-hypnosis to do as a mental exercise. I thought it was amusing and quite comforting, so I used to do it from time to time.

When I read the magazine story, I started to think more clearly. In it, the fertility clinician talked of working with hypnosis to relax patients, and stated that sometimes during hypnosis, subconscious blocks from the past were released, helping people to achieve a pregnancy. While thinking of this, I realised that the problem I had (apart from the physical ones) was that although I really wanted a baby, I couldn't actually picture myself with one. It wasn't real. When I thought about that on the long flight, I realised that although my mother had been told to have no more children after me, I had longed for a baby in the family. I had never dared say anything as it was 'because' of me there couldn't be any. That deep desire for a baby had been there for as long as I could remember, but it was always unfulfilled ... and remained so. I started to use my self-hypnosis a little more, changing the message to try to allow my mind to accept the baby the doctors were working for physically.

The month my son was conceived I had a strong dream of being about seven months pregnant — in the dream I actually stroked my huge, hard stomach. I'd never even touched a pregnant woman's stomach until then. I felt it was a major sign and was fairly certain when my period was late that this time the treatment had worked.

It would be lovely to say I relaxed then and felt assured I'd have a healthy baby. Our avocado tree had its first fruit — just one — right outside the bathroom window. Each time I went to the loo, I was terrified the telltale pink stains would be there and this baby would fall out, too. I told myself the foetus was about the same size as the tiny avocado. If the avocado hung on, so might the baby.

The first scan at the dreaded ultrasound unit showed a heartbeat. I was amazed I could feel happy in the place where I'd had so much heartbreak. It was the best pulsating dot I'd ever seen.

The amniocentesis was another worry — with a slight miscarriage risk. My trusted gynaecologist did the procedure himself, leaving little time for me to panic, just the joy of seeing a tiny, comical sea horse leaping around inside me. It started to be more real.

A few weeks after that, there was a dreaded pink stain on my knickers. I raced off to the clinic filled with fear. A scan showed all was well, but that the placenta was awkwardly placed (placenta praevia), so there was every chance I'd have to have a caesarean birth and it could be premature.

It was never going to be an easy birth as the fibroids were growing apace with the baby. At this point we made the decision that I would take my long-service leave — one of the benefits of being an older mother and having had a career first — and go to our French house and stay as relaxed as possible in the last four months. A referral from a friend to a French clinic in the nearest town produced a very sympathetic and accomplished obstetrician, with all the latest facilities if the baby was premature.

I learned not to look at a fax from my office if it came in the middle of the night — problems there were better dealt with in the morning, rather than spending a sleepless, frustrating night, unable to do anything from such a distance. I didn't dare even buy a baby crib or clothes until I was past the point where they said the foetus was viable. I studied my pregnancy guide book before each doctor's appointment to look up all the possible words in the dictionary beforehand. Schoolgirl French does not equip you for everything! Just to confuse me, the baby pushed through the fibroids and got himself into position for a normal birth. I was appalled. I explained to the doctor that I hadn't done any classes to have a baby normally — never thinking it was an option. The placenta had somehow sorted itself out. He laughed and said something like women have been having babies since long before classes began.

My last major trauma was when the baby stopped moving about a week before the due date. I cried with hopelessness. The doctor assured me he was just a bit cramped, but arranged for me to have foetal heart monitoring every few days in the last week. That thudding, amplified beat was very reassuring.

The day before he was due, the *sage femme* (literally wise woman, but the translation for midwife) told me labour had started, the baby's heart rhythm had changed. We went home and waited; I had time to wash my hair and organise myself.

The fibroids won, and Daniel Jonathan was finally born by caesarean section on 5 August at 16:40. In hospital, he instantly became known as 'le petit Wallaby' — in our Rugby-loving area, he was a kilo bigger than the other babies. He was their first baby born with the aid of a dictionary.

All mothers of these special babies have to deal with additional fears and expectations — and learn to live with them, as discussed in a later chapter. Of course all children are special, but the emotion invested in these babies is perhaps disproportionate. And my French wasn't good enough for me to tell my doctor precisely how hard Daniel was to get.

Soon it was time to go back to Australia and back to work.

I went to visit the nursery Daniel was to attend and, although the matron was great, the big room of iron beds was a bit Dickensian. Then a small blonde toddler started following me around. The matron said, 'It's all right dear, he thinks you are his mother, you look a bit like her.' I just couldn't leave Daniel there. We started trying to juggle — my husband's then freelance work, my job and Daniel.

For the first time I resented my job. I found it scary that I could be at work and hardly think of my baby, I switched back into magazines so entirely. Then other times I'd be stuck in traffic and think of him and suddenly the milk ducts would start to respond. I went to a cosmetic launch luncheon and *Cosmopolitan*'s founding editor, Sylvia Raynor, who'd been sitting opposite me seeing my dress get tighter and tighter, came across and hissed at me to go home and feed that baby. She had gone back to work straight after her baby was born, so she knew.

Sore feet and knees sent me to the doctor and a diagnosis of rheumatoid arthritis. I was appalled. I'd tried so hard to have this baby and now I mightn't be able to play with him or even carry him. At this point, magazines suddenly switched in priority. I felt I'd done what I set out to do in that industry, there was not much further to go, and this baby we'd created seemed much more important. I resigned, invoking the wrath of the previously sympathetic publisher. I was not quite reinvented as a French housewife. After a few months, the arthritis subsided — a clinical study I read a year later showed rheumatoid arthritis can be triggered by a hormone produced by breast feeding.

No other achievement will ever be as total or feel as good as this sturdy little son, hearing him prattling away effortlessly in English or French.

I was one of the lucky ones — many of the other women interviewed for this book haven't ended up with what the clinics sometimes call a 'take-home baby'. Writing the book was prompted by two special friends, both childless. When I started talking to them, asking questions about their problems, answering their questions from my experience, they both kept saying, 'But why didn't someone tell me that?'

Infertility is an isolated and isolating experience. The stigma attached to being barren must come from some deeply buried genetic memory. I reacted angrily one day when a television interviewer made a condescending and factually incorrect assessment of some aspect of infertility. My husband said, 'What are you going to do about it? When will you write your book?'

As I started making notes, it was that sense of isolation I remembered most. While friends and staff were effortlessly having babies, I was stoically covering up my own pain and longing. There was no one I could share my feelings with — even my sister and closest friends couldn't help.

I didn't know about support groups then. Of course, I knew they existed, but I loftily thought I could cope on my own. What a waste. I wish I'd known what a rich source of support and information they could be.

This book taps into the experiences of many people who have had to seek help to have a baby. In the twenty years since the first test-tube baby was born, new reproductive techniques have opened up areas of emotional experience which simply didn't exist before.

All the stages of fertility investigation and treatment are explored, from deciding you may need help, the tests required of both partners and the feelings these tests produce. Facing the results ('I felt I'd been hit on the head with a brick', said one man upon finding his sperm was hopeless), and what the options are, are also covered. Conversations with fellow patients answer the questions about various procedures in assisted conceptions, and also discuss the emotional impact of a pregnancy which doesn't begin in the marital bed.

This isn't a medical encyclopaedia of infertility treatment, it is up to members of the medical profession to write those. Nor does it delve into the various drugs used in assisted reproductive technology, except where quoted by patients in relation to their own treatments. Your fertility specialist is the person to tell you about those, and how they relate to your specific case.

It is, however, a book of rich experiences — those of real people as they have undergone infertility treatment, with the input of many skilled fertility professionals to put those experiences into context. I hope reading it will make the rite of passage into intrusive conception a less lonely one.

Chapter 2
The Myth and Magic
of Assisted Reproduction

'Science moves haphazardly, and often unpredictably. Yet what is merely a gleam
in the eye of a research scientist today may be familiar to everyone tomorrow.'
**Professor Robert Edwards, scientist responsible
for the world's first IVF baby**

'There'll be opposition, I just hope everybody will understand
what we are trying to do and why.'
**Dr Patrick Steptoe, gynaecologist responsible
for the world's first IVF baby**

'Thank you for my baby, thank you.'
Lesley Brown, mother of the world's first IVF baby

Was It Only Twenty Years Ago?

On 25 July 1978 at 11.47 p.m., at Oldham, Lancashire, in northern England, Dr Patrick
Steptoe delivered Louise Joy Brown, the first baby to be born from conception outside
her mother's body. At that moment, the word 'infertile' ceased to be a life sentence.
Hope now lightened the lives of many couples facing the future yearning for a family.

Until then, if you didn't conceive naturally, you didn't have a child. Admittedly, there
were a few ovulation-inducing drugs that were used, some hormone therapies for men
and women. Corrective surgery was sometimes attempted and artificial insemination
was available for those whose problems were related to the male partner. If the woman
had damaged tubes or ovaries, however, there were no options for having your own
child. Adoption (if you qualified) was one solution or perhaps fostering the' illegitimate'
child of another family member. Most families contained special aunts and uncles who
hadn't been able to have children. Childishly canny, you always knew these were the
ones that would give you special attention when your parents were too busy or tired,
these extended parents always managed to have treats tucked away for you, you always
had a good time if you went on holiday with them. If it was spoken about at all in the
family, it was with a twinge of sadness, but a sense of finality.

I had two such aunts and uncles who played special roles in my life. My only
complaint was that one couldn't tie my hair ribbons just the way mum did. Otherwise,

11

we were happy to head off on holiday with them any time. The stories about their child-lessness somehow took on a tragic/romantic note for someone with my imagination.

One, my mother's sister, had had a ruptured appendix when she was a baby, and they stitched her up, as family lore has it, so she could have the family photos taken before she died. A wonderful studio photograph of two golden-ringleted older sisters with a brunette tot propped up between them, captures this moment. All in their white broderie anglaise frills, circa 1910, this was supposed to be the last photo. However, this aunt lived to her full three score years and ten, as she reminded us, but in this clumsy, primitive surgery, her fertility was lost forever.

The other was a great aunt, and a wise and wonderful friend during my teenage traumas. She told me sadly she had had seven miscarriages. I guess now, she could have been diagnosed, given hormones to support the pregnancies, a stitch in the cervix, or whatever else was needed and she may have become a mother. Instead, she adopted my mother in her heart, then me when she came to live near us. As there was no choice then, for women like them, somehow they accepted their lot. Whatever bitterness and sadness they may have felt certainly went into making them into extended parents for us and our contemporaries.

Then, in July 1978, infertility changed forever. I remember the excitement in the office at the *Australian Women's Weekly*. We had bought the rights to the story about the world's first test-tube baby, Louise Brown, born in England as a result of work being done by gynaecologist Dr Patrick Steptoe and embryologist Dr Robert Edwards.

At that time, I was acting Production Editor, and within that role, I had to write the summary of subjects for publicity for the advertising agency and publisher each week. What a brilliant story we had for publicity that week. We all sensed its importance, even me—although fertility was my problem at that stage, not infertility. The subject was full of controversy, too, with doom merchants forecasting the end of procreation (and life) as we knew it.

The whole office was buzzing, as it was literally a case of 'hold the presses' as we waited for the story and photographs to arrive — international pilots were entrusted with this precious cargo in those days before electronic transmissions. Lesley Brown was a young married woman, helping to bring up her husband's child from a previous marriage. She lived in an area with lots of youngish couples, and the maze of prams and pregnant tummies that seem to surround you when you know you can't conceive. She had an operation to try and repair her blocked tubes and was devastated when that hadn't worked. Lesley and her husband John then started to investigate adoption, but found there was a lengthy waiting list and a rigorous and severe selection process.

In despair, Lesley rang the clinic where she had been operated on to repair her tubes. The clinic doctor told them of a specialist who was working with people like them. He worked some distance away, but the doctor said she would write to him on their behalf if they wished.

That doctor was Patrick Steptoe. He had been aware of the tragedy of childlessness since his earliest days as a student doctor when one of the patients asked, 'Doctor, what have I done wrong not to have a family of my own?' During this consultation, the senior specialist explained the workings of her ovaries and tubes to the patient and how her tubes had become blocked, preventing sperm and egg from meeting.

She asked, 'Doctor, can't the Fallopian tubes be by-passed?'

The answer then was a resounding no — sometimes they could be repaired, but never by-passed. Little did Patrick Steptoe then know that he and a young scientist, Dr Robert Edwards, would share that quest.

Now, as patients, we routinely have diagnostic laparoscopies, where the surgeon makes a tiny cut and inserts a small telescope-like instrument with a light into the abdomen inflated with gas and explores and corrects any small defects, but it was Dr Steptoe who pioneered the use of this method in England. Until then, women had to have a laparotomy, major abdominal surgery, just for a diagnosis.

For many years, Dr Steptoe had been frustrated at having to make a full incision to assess a patient's condition, and had wished for a 'safe, efficient way to peer into the abdomen without having to resort to a laparotomy incision'. He had read papers by doctors pioneering methods of exploration, via the vagina, but none of these seemed effective. He then read of a doctor in France, head of an infertility unit at a Paris hospital, inserting a laparoscope, an instrument that worked like a telescope, into the abdomen at the navel.

He discovered that, if the abdomen was filled with harmless gas, the method worked. The difficulty, however, was that the electric lamp in the apparatus quickly became hot, so they had to work with utmost speed. In Germany, a doctor backed by a lens-manufacturing company showed him a film, revealing a more sophisticated laparoscope than the one used in Paris.

Dr Steptoe was given support from his Hospital Management Committee to buy the new German equipment. He then began practising (not on live patients to begin with) until he had perfected the technique and was ready to perform laparoscopies on live patients. Meanwhile, French scientists improved the equipment further and, with a new quartz rod, an intense light could be distributed, cooled by a fan outside the body, so that colour photographs of the condition were possible for permanent records.

In 1967, Dr Steptoe was to publish the first textbook on the use of laparoscopy in gynaecology, hoping to convince his sceptical colleagues of the benefits of this new diagnostic tool. He was working out of the mainstream in a regional hospital at Oldham, in northern England, and it was his expertise in using a laparoscope that drew him to the attention of Dr Robert Edwards, a scientist who had been working on the fertilisation of eggs outside the human body.

Dr Edwards knew he could progress no further in helping childless couples unless there was a relatively non-traumatic method of collecting the eggs from the female ovary, one not requiring major surgery. Dr Steptoe's laparoscopies seemed to be the answer. He telephoned him from his lab in Cambridge, following it up with a meeting at a medical conference. So began a long association, requiring frequent trips up and down Great Britain.

Dr Edwards had begun university studying agriculture, but switched to zoology, finding the scientific study of reproduction in animals more interesting than that of plants. After his doctorate, he worked with a colleague, using hormones to trigger the release of multiple eggs in mice for fertilisation.

Edwards said: 'It was like setting accurate alarm clocks. Give the hormones at midday and then at midnight the clamour of bells would all begin together. What happened to the eggs in that 12-hour interval [after the injection of serum from the urine of pregnant women]?' Edwards and his colleague began examining the eggs under a microscope.

After a year in California, Dr Edwards returned to England and worked at the department of Experimental Biology at Mill Hill, North London. Although working on immunology, he was still drawn to embryology. Having had children effortlessly with his wife Ruth, he was drawn to the plight of some childless friends, making him wonder for the first time about replanting human embryos in a woman's womb. He began exploring the possibilities of working on human eggs, and found their own obstetrician was willing to part with surplus ovarian tissue after surgical procedures.

After unsuccessful attempts at ripening eggs, he suddenly theorised that perhaps human eggs took longer than rodents and, sure enough, this proved correct as he watched the first egg ripening. He then theorised that if the egg could ripen in vitro (literally 'in glass' — a Petri dish or test-tube), perhaps it could be fertilised in vitro, providing a means for sperm and egg to meet where this was impossible inside the woman's body. He knew, however, that this technique would arouse hostility. Even the ethical issues surrounding donor insemination aroused hostility then. When a new head of the department joined and was opposed to in vitro fertilisation (IVF) on ethical grounds, Edwards eventually left and rejoined his former head at the Physiological Laboratory in Cambridge, working both on immunology and embryology.

At about this time, in 1968, Dr Steptoe and Dr Edwards finally met. It was to take ten years of constant work, however, before the first baby was born using their techniques. First the fluid in which the eggs were to ripen and fertilise had to be perfected. Then the woman's hormone dosage and timing had to be finely tuned to stimulate the egg ripening. Also, the egg had to be removed at the right moment. An instrument to suck out the minute egg had to be devised, plus another to replace the fertilised embryo in the uterus.

Dr Edwards explained his view of developing life, in the face of all the opposition they were facing in their work, as follows: 'The beginnings of life have never failed to fascinate me. It is a period rich and strange in change and movement. The microscopic embryonic cells move elegantly and precisely along their appointed pathway, forming a succession of shapes before they emerge into the pattern of their human form.'

Dr Edwards had, by this stage, found a suitable fluid in which the egg and sperm would mix and fertilise, but it took many years before Edwards and Dr Steptoe were sure the resulting conception was suitable for replacement in a mother's womb. When they did reach that stage, they were swamped with volunteers from Dr Steptoe's childless patients. Among them were Lesley and John Brown.

After an initial diagnostic laparoscopy, Lesley Brown had her damaged tubes removed. She then reported each time her period started to Dr Steptoe, as he'd explained to her that timing was critical.

She went and stayed at a small cottage hospital near Oldham, where Dr Steptoe worked, and an egg was removed. The doctor called two days later and told her they were going to replace the egg, fertilised with her husband's sperm, in her uterus that afternoon. They delayed the procedure for a few more hours until the egg became more fully developed, and finally replaced it at midnight.

Lesley Brown described every day after that as a day of hope for her. At the time, she and her husband didn't realise the treatment was in such a pioneering phase. She thought IVF was openly available to everyone.

Initially, tubal surgery had been seen as the only answer for women such as Lesley, and some doctors had success in this field. Tubal transplants were also tried — from donors — and artificial tubes. The donor tubes were technically possible, but the drugs required to prevent rejection of transplanted tissue were very toxic.

Professor Carl Wood, the Australian pioneer of infertility treatment, was not far behind in the race to have the world's first IVF baby. In fact, the first IVF pregnancy was credited to his team in Melbourne in 1973. It resulted in early embryo death, but at last the doctors knew the technique could work.

Professor Wood had become aware of work with sheep's embryos in New South Wales, and the possibility of donor embryo transfer in humans was suggested. IVF became a better option, however, as the egg would belong to the woman, not a donor, and the sperm to her husband. Still, IVF or embryo transfer had still not been achieved in larger animals, only in mice. In the early 1970s, Professor Wood assembled a team which worked towards changing the lives of the infertile, training a physiologist Alex Lopata as a specialist embryologist as there was no one locally available with appropriate training. Professor Wood said that, in Australia, the pressure was really on doctors to aid infertile couples. Since the advent of the contraceptive pill and the slight loosening of abortion laws, the number of babies available for adoption was becoming fewer and fewer.

'The first baby born at our clinic was in 1980,' said Professor Wood. 'This was the result of the development of IVF in Melbourne by a combined team at Monash and Melbourne Universities [Professor Wood was Chairman of the group]. The research commenced in 1970, one or two years after Bobby Edwards and Patrick Steptoe in the United Kingdom. We did have the first IVF pregnancy in 1973, which was published in the *Lancet*, the medical journal, but it only lasted 1–2 weeks and it was not for another seven years [that] we had our first baby. Naturally I was very pleased and relieved at the baby's birth. Our initial anxieties were mainly related to the safety of the technique as the reassuring evidence in mouse and hamster was that no abnormalities would occur. However, we can never be completely sure that what applies to one species would apply to another. It was not until more than 100 babies were born at our clinic that I began to relax concerning the safety of the technique as far as the baby is concerned.'

IVF or 'assisted reproductive technology', as it is more correctly called, progressed beyond anyone's dreams in its first twenty years. Now a baby of their own would seem to be at least a possibility (although not a probability yet) for all infertile couples. The knowledge and techniques extend well beyond the original concept of helping women with blocked tubes. Patients with all kinds of infertility can benefit from the intense scrutiny of early human life which has been a direct result of IVF technology. The ethics debate along the way, however, has been almost as difficult as the work itself.

The idea of a baby starting its life in a test-tube or Petri dish, not within its mother's body, was emotive stuff, and it seemed everyone had an opinion about the morality of such a thing. From church leader to politician, everyone seemed to find some objection. People spoke of space age stuff, brave new world experimentation on babies' lives, all fed via a greedy-for-controversy media.

One of the most traumatic aspects of Louise Brown's birth was trying to keep the media away from the hospital, and nothing has changed since then. The only people who didn't object were the infertile. For them, at last, there was some hope.

Even now, governments seem to meddle in the lives of the infertile in a way they wouldn't dare with the normally fertile. Professor Wood comments: 'I do think governments have intruded too much in IVF technology. The ill effects of natural conception on children as the result of parents conceiving when they smoke or take excessive alcohol, which may adversely affect the baby, or not having Rubella (German measles) immunisation are a much more serious risk to the offspring than any possible side-effects of IVF technology. I think governments have been oversensitive because of research done during World War II by the Nazi groups on humans and the encouragement of the Nazi political system to breed people of a particular physical type. Medicine in most countries has a system for checking the legal and ethical basis of medical procedures. In my state, Victoria, there are statutes controlling IVF which make a large bureaucracy within the government and use a lot of money which would be better used somewhere else in the health system. I have more than forty-two consent forms for patients on the IVF program. In the same city, one needs only one consent form to have a heart transplant!'

Within all the excitement of Dr Steptoe's dream of a day when every woman can have a baby of her own, there is the reality of the statistics.

The human species is not very fertile. Only around 20 per cent of normally fertile couples conceive in a cycle where they have tried to do so and timed everything to perfection. Statistics within fertility treatment are impossible to quote, such is the variation from clinic to clinic, from patient to patient, with factors such as age and physical problems needing to be built into the equation. They vary between 10 per cent and 30 per cent, depending on which statistics you see.

Every couple *has* to believe they will conceive immediately they start on a program of assisted fertility. They believe they will be the exception, defying the statistics. It is bewildering, as a patient, to find you haven't conceived when your hormones have been monitored daily to pinpoint ovulation, ovulation has been seen on a scan, or evidence of it has been shown from raised hormone levels. You know the good sperm and egg were placed together at the same time. So why doesn't it work every time?

That is the big question confronting patients and doctors alike. Why do patients with poor chances of conception miraculously conceive normally? Why do those with very good chances and no evident problems fail to do so? How does the embryo select its site to implant in the uterus? Why does it very often not find a site and disappear with the menstrual flow? Is it the Creator's private joke?

Many milestones have been passed in infertility treatment. Each year treatment is further refined, breakthroughs are made. The breakthrough of the 1990s has been the technique of micro-injecting sperm into the centre of the woman's egg. This has changed the lives of many couples whose male partner had major sperm deficiencies. This treatment is called ICSI (pronounced ik-sy) or intracytoplasmic sperm injection. It means that if a man produces any good sperm at all, this technique can be attempted, using IVF technology for egg collection and embryo replacement in the woman. Up until this technique was pioneered, donor sperm or adoption was considered the only alternative. With improved surgical techniques, even immature sperm can be aspirated from within the testes and used in this way.

What has changed about the techniques involving test-tube babies in this first twenty years? And what can really be done, and what can rarely be done? The confusion about what is and is not possible arises because the more sensational cases are often the ones reported.

~

'If it's newsworthy, it means it's uncommon and people don't see that, and consequently they develop unreal expectations. They think medicine can do anything. Panic hits women at about the age of 37, and sadly, some doctors aren't aware of this panic as they potter along at their own speed and the patient becomes more and more agitated.'
Dr Stephen J. Steigrad, Director of the Department of Reproductive Medicine at the Royal Hospital for Women, Randwick, NSW, Australia

The other day my sister casually mentioned a friend who is having fertility treatment and she said that the sperm retrieved from the friend's husband hadn't been good, and that her eggs were not able to be frozen. I commented that, as far as I knew, egg freezing hadn't been perfected yet; only a minute number of babies had been born following egg freezing as the loss rate at thawing was great. However, because my sister had seen a news story about these successful cases, she assumed that all egg freezing was quite straightforward now.

And therein lies the danger. Because of the number of stories we all read about successful or bizarre treatments, they seem commonplace. Somehow, we assume any 60-year-old grandmother can enter a fertility program and, with the aid of a donated egg and hormone therapy, have a successful pregnancy. We assume that sperm and eggs and embryos all thaw successfully and can be reclaimed the moment the whim takes us for an instant pregnancy.

In all the reporting about the case of a woman in England trying to gain permission to use her dead husband's frozen sperm to create a baby, no one ever asked the question about whether the sperm had survived the freezing, and whether the woman would be someone who fell pregnant easily or someone who needed many cycles to conceive — cycles for which she may not have had enough sperm. Or even if she could conceive at all. In common discussion, it was assumed she would be pregnant the minute the court gave the word. This happens perhaps because news stories are often notoriously brief, and the terms and procedures in assisted conception are both complicated and confusing. So the details are simply left out most of the time.

A similar situation occurred when an English woman was carrying nine foetuses after hormone therapy. It was sensational. The doctors were portrayed as monsters for suggesting that the number of foetuses should be reduced — i.e. some should be destroyed — to allow a greater chance of her giving birth to some of her babies. She miscarried them all. Without giving the details, the stories suggested that doctors were irresponsible in allowing this pregnancy to happen. Only one report showed that the woman had been told that her ovaries were becoming overstimulated with the fertility drugs she was taking and that she should abandon trying to become pregnant that cycle and avoid intercourse.

Abandoned cycles are quite common during infertility treatment. Not only can overstimulated ovaries require hospitalisation, but doctors also know that there is a high chance of a multiple pregnancy rate and a low chance of these babies developing to full term and being safely born. In the news stories, it was implied that the doctors were doing something very wrong. The truth is that they are now either very regulated (the United Kingdom) or strictly self-regulated (Australia) to replace no more than three embryos after a cycle of IVF, thus avoiding more than triplets, which have a better survival rate.

News stories about assisted reproduction continue to make the headlines. Why? Is it that they are a combination of human tragedy, hope and quasi-sexual titillation? The perfect tabloid mix.

The cloning of Dolly the sheep in Scotland sent shivers of fear around the world as politicians and the news media speculated on the ramifications of cloning for humans and the likelihood that science fiction films and Hitler's eugenics experiments were not just medical aberrations.

The shivers became more intense when an American physicist, Dr Richard Seed, announced his plans to set up the first human cloning clinic, modifying the methods used for Dolly the sheep. He announced in January 1998 that he could take an unfertilised egg from a woman's ovary, remove the egg's nucleus, and replace it with the nucleus of an adult cell taken from either of the parents or a third party. Thus a child could be the identical twin of its parents, but several decades younger.

The American Society for Reproductive Medicine, which sets ethical standards for reproductive medicine in the USA for its members, said human cloning was unacceptable and it called for a voluntary five-year moratorium while further animal and DNA research was carried out.

In the United Kingdom, a law was passed in 1990 banning human cloning. A recent World Medical Association meeting in Hamburg, Germany, also made a unanimous call for doctors to stop working in this field until all its ramifications are considered. The call was supported by doctors from seventy countries (more than five million doctors) representing a wide range of cultures and religions.

What is the reality of assisted reproduction? And the future?

All the experts agree the one thing they cannot fix is maternal egg age. They all state that when a woman reaches the age of around 38, the quality of her eggs declines rapidly. So even if a pregnancy does occur, there is a rate of around 30 per cent early pregnancy loss. Contrary to the demands of our career/consumer society and the concept of women's liberation, maternal egg age is one immoveable barrier to life on our terms. We may have come a long way, baby — the slogan of the 1970s — but not that far!

Dr Steigrad comments:

I think we are losing track of things. We have become too commercially oriented, far more interested in acquiring things, so people put off child bearing while they achieve goals. Then they say now we'll have a baby and they find age has passed them by. Women do have better places in the workforce, managerial roles, greater opportunities than existed, so they get an opportunity to be head of a department, an increase in salary, travel, and they put their career ahead of forming a relationship. I see many more couples in their late thirties now who have only been married a short time. That's a pattern we didn't see before. There is no formal upper age limit for treatment, but we get very edgy at the age of 40, because we know the chances are so poor, and we counsel patients with that in mind. Their chances of conception in a single cycle are down to single digits. There are some clinics who used to have an age limit of 38, but now it is 40 or 42. Certainly conceptions after that age are very rare. And the early pregnancy loss rate is staggeringly high. So it is not good for the patients and not good for the clinic staff. And after that there is still pre-natal diagnosis to get through [to check for any abnormalities].

Professor Robert Jansen, of Sydney IVF, adds: 'Age-related infertility in the woman is the most frustrating diagnosis. Anything else is manageable. We don't arbitrarily close doors, but in practice, 42 is usually the upper limit for a GIFT cycle [where tubes are clear and egg and sperm are surgically placed in the tube, hoping for fertilisation] and 40 for IVF.'

I feel education of women must be more thorough. I had not seen or read anything about egg age when I took my first step into a fertility clinic. I had been in journalism since I was 16, and had read everything I could get my hands on about fertility and later infertility. I truly thought the doctors tried to encourage us to have children earlier because of other physical factors — such as our bodies being more malleable when we are younger and to avoid conditions such as high blood pressure in pregnancy. And I dismissed most of this as being old-fashioned nonsense, reasoning that women were much younger and fitter now in their late 30s than ever before, so the doctors had it wrong. I thought that as long as the eggs were still being produced, they would function well until the time they finally ceased in menopause. It would have certainly startled me if I had realised that in pursuing my career so enthusiastically, thinking I had all the time in the world, I was flirting with the death of my fertility.

'One of the most common myths of patients is that if they stay fit they stay fertile,' said Professor Jansen.

Professor Ian Craft at the London Fertility Centre confirms that he is also seeing a lot of women in their late 30s or early 40s who have delayed starting a family while they pursued their career goals. He stated: 'It usually comes as a great shock when I inform them their chances of conceiving become significantly less as they get older. In my view, this is a public education issue. We need to teach people the biology of conception.'

In a recent television interview, he added that he thought nature should be a guideline to the age at which doctors will stop helping women become mothers. In his view, women can conceive naturally up until the age of fifty-five, and therefore it is appropriate to help them up until that age.

British reproductive biology specialist Professor Roger Gosden asserts: 'We must remember that deferring fertility is a gamble. Journalists and broadcasters are probably in a better position than doctors to raise public awareness of this under-acknowledged fact of biology.'

Are There Any Negative Aspects Following Fertility Treatment?

Disappointment is the key one, because even using an optimistic success rate of 20 per cent per cycle; in one hundred women, it still means eighty of those will end up without a baby.

Most clinics and hospitals are carefully monitoring the responses of patients to the hormone therapy both during and after IVF treatment. In a study carried out by Monash IVF (Victoria, Australia) following up 10 358 women registered with the clinic between 1978 and 1992, results showed that women on this program showed no increased incidence of breast cancer or ovarian cancer.

Women on the program were shown to have a significantly higher incidence of uterine cancer, but this included women who had not been exposed to fertility drugs, as well as those who had. Women with unexplained infertility had a significantly higher risk of ovarian and uterine cancer, whether or not they were exposed to fertility drugs, than the general population.

As these treatments are at most 20 years old, statistics are still very new. Longer term studies of cancer-incidence after infertility and IVF are necessary. The researchers are conducting another similar study of more than 30 000 women from fertility clinics all around Australia to provide further information.

While I was doing the research for this book, it occurred to me that if women begin life with a certain number of eggs in their ovaries, and expect to lose just one each cycle, will the hyper-stimulation of their ovaries and the harvesting of multiple eggs in a cycle affect the duration of their years before menopause? I asked Professor Wood.

'We do not know the answer,' he said. 'It has been considered that the extra eggs used each month would not bring on an early menopause, but this will only be determined when the couples have been followed up on after menopause. Such studies are in progress.'

What Is the Future of Assisted Reproductive Technology?

Most doctors agree that the way forward is refinement of currently used techniques and hormones, coupled with a far greater understanding of early embryonic life.

In their book *Infertility: All Your Questions Answered*, Professor Carl Wood and Professor Gab Kovacs predict that pre-conception diagnosis will become increasingly possible, which will help couples with genetic disease. At the moment, these tests are carried out once the pregnancy is established, requiring a termination of the pregnancy if the test shows an abnormality is present.

Embryo biopsy would allow minuscule cells to be tested before the embryo is replaced into the mother, and only embryos free of the disorder would be replaced.

Professor Jansen, when asked what he would advise a young woman today if she knew she wanted a baby at some time in her life, replied: 'It sounds a bit twenty-first century, but consider a laparoscopy, a biopsy of the ovary and the storage of the removed tissue (and its eggs) for insurance.'

Dr Steigrad comments:

We are refining all the time. We can now get sperm out of the testes by needle biopsy, immature sperm, and it works. I think we'll see a lot more of IVF being involved with embryo biopsy in couples where there is a known genetic problem. We'll be able to select out the embryos that carry that problem. I'm not talking about building a super-race, we'll save a lot of emotional pain if we only implant those embryos that are normal. We must also work on the freezing of eggs without the appalling loss rate. The other thing we will be looking at is the freezing of ovarian tissue, pre-follicle forming (and ovulation). I don't like the idea of freezing ovarian tissue for the woman who plans to delay child bearing till her late 40s, I think that is an abuse of the technology, but I am sure it will be done. But in the case of a woman who is going to have treatment for cancer, it would help enormously. Once we learn to freeze eggs effectively, we won't need to freeze

REGULATIONS — WHO DECIDES?

As Professor Carl Wood, the Melbourne fertility pioneer, states, governments have generally become more involved in regulating infertility treatments than most other areas of medicine probably as a result of public outrage at Nazi experiments carried out in the death camps during World War II. However, excessive caution can lead to inflexible laws.

There is continuing debate around the world between those who think self-regulation by the ethics committees of the medical profession is more appropriate and those who prefer specific government legislation controlling new treatments and technologies. Essentially, the discussion centres on whether infertility is a medical or a social problem. And whether governments or the patient's medical adviser should determine appropriate medical treatments.

In the United Kingdom, such a law was introduced in 1990 and a governing body created to administer that law. This body is called the Human Fertilisation and Embryology Authority (HFEA), and since 1991 all fertility centres have been licensed and subject to annual inspection and licence renewal. The HFEA publishes an annual report and a patients' guide giving results at fertility clinics around the country; these are available at no cost from the HFEA. The National Health Service regional authorities have widely differing funding allocated for infertility patients. Private treatment is expensive, and most British couples do not have private health insurance.

In Australia, there is no federal law controlling fertility treatment. Some individual states have specific laws relating to assisted reproductive technology, but the overall national policy is governed by the federal council of the Fertility Society of Australia, which includes a consumer representative as well as medical practitioners. This self-regulation in accordance with Australian medical research and ethics protects patients and also ensures that clinics are providing correct services. The general feeling is that government legislation is difficult to change. Even the most well-intentioned laws can quickly prove obsolete in such a rapidly changing field as assisted reproductive technology (ART). The British tradition of medical ethics applies to issues such as the donation, not sale, of eggs, sperm and embryos.

Looking at fertility treatment internationally, the Australian system — where Medicare (the national public health system) covers six cycles of stimulated IVF-type procedures in a woman's lifetime — is considered generous, although doctors and patients question the arbitrary cut-off point for public health cover.

In the United States, the American Society for Reproductive Medicine publishes minimum standards for assisted reproductive technologies and all members are expected to follow these voluntary standards. Guidelines are offered on issues dealing with donor eggs or sperm, and screening, testing and medical techniques. There, however, the similarity to the Australian situation ends.

The American Bill of Rights guarantees unrestricted trade — incorporating selling and advertising. This allows the sale of 'donated' eggs, sperm and embryos, and the advertising of clinics to carry out ART. The United States medical insurance system is limited and only recently have various courts in the USA accepted that infertility is a 'disease' claimable on medical insurance. Even so, many insurance companies severely limit treatment, so only one cycle a year may be attempted. There are almost no fertility units providing IVF for non-paying patients.

In New Zealand, a private member's Bill was introduced in 1997 to attempt to regulate infertility services, with criminal penalties and legal prohibitions threatened within it. Neither this Bill nor a more general government Bill has yet become law, leaving physician self-regulation in place. Public funding for fertility treatment is severely rationed, covering only about 50 per cent of costs for infertility treatment and availability depends on where you live.

Semen is now for sale on the Internet, challenging international laws and ethics on the sale of human gametes. In the United Kingdom, the HFEA is investigating this practice, although it is unclear how gametes, once purchased, can be transported from one country to another. Technology — both in assisted reproduction and cyberspace — is again testing the legislators.

embryos. When you are dealing with sperm you are dealing in millions, lose a million here or there and it doesn't matter. But if you can withdraw nine eggs in a woman, then eliminate the ones that aren't good quality, then lose a third of them in the thawing, it isn't great odds. The problem with embryo freezing is that the woman may not have chosen her partner yet or it may be inappropriate with her medical condition to stimulate her to get eggs. But to take pieces of ovary, we can do that very quickly, whereas it may take a couple of months to organise a stimulation cycle of hormones, and there may not be time. Finally, the patient must understand all aspects of it, including the down side, that makes life much easier for us. No unreal expectations!

A new development has just been announced by Monash IVF, suggesting a medical breakthrough within IVF treatment. Professor Alan Trounson, from the group, said the new method involves allowing an embryo to develop in vitro for up to three days longer than in conventional methods. This means scientists are better able to gauge which embryos are viable, meaning fewer failures of implantation once they are replaced in the mother's womb. This extra time before replacement better mimics the natural conditions, where an embryo usually spends up to five days in the Fallopian tubes before it reaches the uterus.

These extra days of development have been made possible by the development of a new fluid in which the embryo can continue to develop. Up until now, the culture fluids had not supported life for this length of time, and the use of cultured tubal cells from a donor woman or from animal cells is restricted in Australia because of the risk of disease transmission or other illnesses. Other fertility clinics from around the world are greeting this breakthrough with scientific caution, but also with the hope that it will fulfil the initial promise of doubling IVF success rates.

Have Community Attitudes
Changed in This First Twenty Years?

Unfortunately, probably not, or not in fundamental ways.

Unless someone is touched by infertility personally, empathy is rare. Watching a television debate last night about surrogacy, the following crass cliches came spouting out from everyone not intimately involved in infertility:

- World overpopulation—yet how do unwanted babies in the Third World materialise in a child-deprived household of the West, particularly when inter-country adoption laws are mostly prohibitive?
- The abortion rate — again, how do these aborted, unwanted foetuses magically transfer themselves into a waiting, eager uterus?
- Public health service money should be spent on those people who are 'really ill' — ignoring the fact that medical conditions are usually responsible for infertility, and these medical conditions can often be treated. Someone in need of a hip replacement is hardly 'really ill', but their discomfort is real enough. Who has the right to decide which medical conditions are 'really serious'?

Surely if a treatment exists for a medical condition it should be available.

The idea that infertility is some God-given curse to be endured is still prevalent in our society. Not much has changed since biblical days. Enlightenment and emotional recognition of another's pain is the only way forward, to merge the doctors' skills and the public perceptions.

Sandra Dill AM, Executive President of ACCESS, Australia's national infertility awareness group, sums up: 'Most people don't know what to say about infertility. Isn't it curious? Even someone like me, who has had years of IVF treatment and now works full-time in this field. In the customs hall when I was travelling to a conference, the customs officer asked what I did for a living, and I am ashamed to admit I was embarrassed to tell him. How do I tell him I am a consumer advocate for infertile people? So I muttered something about being a manager and fled. I thought about it and I thought: You are out there, going overseas to give talks, you're telling consumers to be more assertive, so they are more open about it, then you can't even tell a customs man, who doesn't give a hang, what you do.

'The next time I said I was a consumer advocate in a medical field, the field of IVF and infertility. I didn't want to hit him over the head with it. It was a man at the desk and he said "Oh," and he looked at me for a minute. I said, "It's OK, it's not catching," and we laughed and moved on.

'But even there, in that line of people, he didn't know what to say. I think that underscores the fact that infertility is [still] a taboo subject. People feel they just don't know what to say.'

Chapter 3
The Wonder of Conception

'It is just an amazing event. It's a constant wonder that it ever actually works.'
Dr Stephen Steigrad, Director, Reproductive Medicine,
Royal Hospital for Women, Randwick, NSW, Australia

~

'As a fertility scientist running a donor insemination clinic, I soon realised
there was more to conceiving than eggs and sperm and tubes and hormones;
that there were subtle physical factors controlling fertility that were not
always detectable by standard investigative approaches.'
Paul Entwistle, Director of the Rodney Clinic, Liverpool, England

For most of us, the scant knowledge we have about conception comes from trying to avoid it. I was absolutely sure the first month I had my intra-uterine device removed I'd be pregnant — why not, I'd been pregnant before, my husband already had a son.

When this doesn't happen, we actually begin to look into the more subtle workings of our bodies. I was forced to become a little more knowledgeable about my fertility than most of my contemporaries because I couldn't take the contraceptive pill, but even so, I didn't know much more than the basics. I could make and read my temperature chart — and that was it. It matched the 'classic' ones in any gynaecological books I had, so I assumed I was ovulating. But as my cycles varied between 21 and 26 days, working out ovulation time in advance was tricky, especially as we both had jobs that could take us away from home.

While trying to avoid conception, I had once read a book called *The Billings Method* about reading your mucus to gauge fertile times, but I could never really get the hang of it. It wasn't until I began at the fertility clinic that the real wonder of it became apparent. In my impatience, I was trying to suggest to the clinic sister that I should be given a fertility drug to guarantee and pinpoint ovulation. It was lesson number one for me. It was calmly explained to me that nature knew best, and if ovulation-inducing drugs could be avoided, they would be, as they could adversely affect the cervical mucus. It hadn't occurred to me that the texture of the cervical mucus played such a critical role and that drug therapy could disturb that.

So my lessons began.

The first day at the clinic at Sydney's Royal Hospital for Women, the sister took out a big chart. She explained how they 'scored' patients to assess their ovulation. She told me that blood tests would be taken each day, before, during and after ovulation, to check my hormone levels. Now oestrogen and progesterone were fairly familiar terms, the common female hormones and ones I had heard about while taking the experimental contraceptive pills. But I also started to learn a new vocabulary which included something mysterious to me called FSH, which I later found out was *follicle stimulating hormone*, which, as its name suggests, stimulates several follicles (like mini-volcanoes on the ovaries), one of which becomes dominant and from which the egg will emerge. Then LH levels were casually discussed. These I discovered were *luteinizing hormones*, which the ovary can detect and which set ovulation in motion. She also explained that samples of cervical mucus would be taken through a speculum each morning during this period to assess what was happening.

She then referred to her big chart to show me what the mucus looked like through a microscope and how the 'ferning' at ovulation time helped the sperm get to the right place at the right time, suitably perky. I saw the first phase which looked like bubbly mineral water, the second phase which looked like condensation running down a window pane, then the critical fishbone-fern formations at ovulation which help the sperm swim up into the uterus and tubes. She then explained that they would check my levels of the hormone progesterone in the last half of the cycle, to make sure the levels were high enough to support a pregnancy if it happened.

Even that amount of information was complex enough, but during that first month at the clinic, patients were invited to a lecture by the doctor in charge of reproductive medicine, Dr Stephen Steigrad, to give us a more specific description of the workings of our bodies. About fifty of us, some couples, some women alone, sat around waiting to have our infertility miraculously explained and overturned.

After the lecture, like most present, I was filled with awe that conception *ever* took place, so many tiny chain reactions were necessary to amount to a successful conception and pregnancy. He began by telling us about ovulation, then the whole conception reaction. Following is a slightly simplified version of Dr Steigrad's lecture:

OVULATION

A woman is born with all the eggs she's ever going to have in her ovaries. She is born with roughly two million eggs. By the time she reaches puberty, she is down to about 200 000–300 000 eggs. Women don't just lose one egg per cycle. Eggs die all the time, unrelated to the menstrual cycle.

In each cycle, women germinate a number of primordial follicles (sites from which the eggs erupt). This may range from three to thirty. One of them will become dominant and the rest will die, so there is a very large rate of egg loss all the time. (Mature follicles have been likened to button mushrooms in appearance, varying from 1.5 to 2.5 cm in diameter.) Therefore, the ovaries have a finite number of eggs to produce and then they run out, and that's the menopause.

There is an assumption that a woman ovulates every month. She doesn't. She can have a menstrual cycle without ovulating. The egg is only a cell and it can die in the follicle before it ruptures (and is released for fertilisation). Another assumption is that when a follicle forms it is going to rupture; it doesn't have to. There is yet another an assumption that the egg will be normal, and it may not be. Umpteen times with IVF treatment we get empty zones, that means an egg shell with no egg, or we get a degenerating egg, or an egg that is too immature. This happens all the time, but more often as part of the ageing process.

THE TUBES

A woman has two Fallopian tubes, extending from the upper section of her uterus. When ovulation takes place, the Fallopian tube has to move across to that portion of the ovary where the follicle is going to rupture and we don't understand how it knows to do that.

The Fallopian tube is not like a vacuum cleaner — it actually embraces that portion of the follicle so the follicle ruptures (the egg) into the Fallopian tube. Anything that interferes with the tubal movement or acts as a barrier between the ovary and the tube is going to prevent conception occurring. Adhesions (the fine strands of scar tissue that form between unconnected parts of internal organs, perhaps as a result of earlier surgery) or endometriosis (where parts of the endometrium, lining of the womb, escape and locate themselves in other parts of the pelvic cavity) can be inhibitors.

The tubes themselves must be clear of blockages. Books usually draw the tubes from the outside, where there is quite a thick muscular wall. Inside there is not very much room, it is as fine as buttonhole thread. I think what people must realise is that the tube is not a piece of PVC piping. It is a living, moving thing, an organ in itself.

THE SPERM

The analysis of semen must be done in a specialist laboratory as the accuracy of semen counts can vary from lab to lab. If the initial tests are done by the GP, then they should send the semen to a reputable laboratory so tests don't have to be repeated when couples come to a fertility clinic.

The technical ease with which a semen analysis is done has been modified over the years with the invention of counting chambers, which has made it much more accurate. But the training of seminologists has become quite labour intensive and there are very few really good ones around. Therefore you have to be incredibly cautious about counts from other than recognised laboratories.

There is a French organisation which has been involved in collecting sperm from around France in the establishment of their national donor insemination program, and they state they are seeing more than a 2 per cent reduction in sperm counts per year. (This echoes other studies in Denmark and Edinburgh.) So if that continues, all men will be azoospermic (have nil sperm) by the year 2050. Admittedly we are seeing it in infertile couples, but we are probably rejecting more sperm donors than before.

There is no question that males are incredibly fragile. And a lot of things do adversely affect sperm counts. It's hard to say specifically which have the most effect. It may be the increased wearing of jockey-type underpants, it may be that in more sedentary occupations the testicles are warmer than they were in past times.

Certainly emotional stress does play a role — particularly in some men, not all. The sperm count varies enormously from week to week in a male, with a big variation on what is normal. There have been studies with students that have shown that as they get closer to their final exams, their sperm counts become poorer and poorer, and frankly some go into the infertile range. Then after the exams they recover again, so it is hard to say. I am guessing there may be something in these reports of declining sperm counts, but the causes are unexplained at this point.

Now, the healthy sperm's role in conception. First, the sperm has to be ejaculated into the female genital tract. The sperm then have to pass through the cervical mucus during which process they undergo or they initiate a process of activation and capacitation and this continues as they travel down the uterus and down the Fallopian tubes.

Roughly half will go down the wrong Fallopian tube (the one that isn't on egg pick-up duty that month). Those that choose the right tube have to reach the end of the Fallopian tube and be there in adequate numbers, having been adequately activated and capacitated, to meet the egg, which we hope has been properly ovulated. They then have to surround the egg like a corona of sperm, releasing enzymes to try to erode the egg shell. The moment one of them does that, gets its head through and makes contact with the egg membrane, then another process takes place, there is a big calcium flux, and that seems to stop any other sperm getting through. The membrane then breaks down between the head of the sperm and the cytoplasm (inner contents) of the egg. The sperm head contents, which are primarily chromosomes, pass into the egg and it forms what we call a pronucleus, the egg nucleus forms the other pronucleus and the fertilisation process continues.

FERTILISATION

Fertilisation takes 24 hours, it doesn't just happen in an instant. The next thing that happens is that the two pronucleii break up, the membranes around them break down and the chromosomes line up. At that point it is called a zygote. It has gone from being a two-cell to a one-cell object and the first division takes place. We now have two blastomeres and a pre-embryo. The division of blastomeres continues until about the eight-cell stage. You can literally take a blastomere away at that stage — and this is what they are doing now with embryo biopsy in lower animals — you can literally keep dividing the embryo and keep creating clones, or twinning. They are absolutely identical as they come from the same blastomere. You can do this up to the eight-cell stage; beyond that, some of the blastomeres take on certain functions.

While all that is happening, the embryo is starting to move down along the Fallopian tube.

IMPLANTATION

On day five, it passes through the junction between tube and uterus into the uterine cavity. Now the uterine cavity is not a cavity at all. When you look at it from the side it is like your two hands pressed together. The walls are in contact, separated by a thin layer of endometrial fluid.

The morula (developing embryo) passes into the uterine cavity at the same time as it becomes a blastocyst—it develops a little puddle of fluid to one side and at this stage, for the first time, you have two different cell types. You have the outer ring of cells which will become the placenta and the membranes, and a small pod of cells to one side called the inner cell mass which will form the embryo. If that doesn't happen, you have something called the *empty sac syndrome* — there is no embryo inside. (A positive pregnancy test will be achieved, but eventually the body will recognise that there is no foetus inside and the pregnancy will spontaneously abort.)

On day five, the blastocyst hatches; up until then it is within its shell. At this point the shell has to break and the blastocyst has to come out of its shell and be free. The pregnancy hormone that it was producing is released into the fluid in the endometrial cavity, and it is now, for the first time, that it can be detected.

The uterus is a muscular organ, and as it contracts, it sets up swirls of fluid — in the same way you get swirls of fluid if you place two pieces of glass together with water in between then press them.

The blastocyst is actually being pushed all over the place while it is developing and growing. On about day seven, the implantation site is selected. We don't know how that happens. Some part of the endometrium (womb lining) becomes better situated for implantation or is more attractive. We don't know why, as the embryo can't move of its own volition. Somehow it has arrived at this site.

Between days eight and ten is probably the implantation window, and that is the time it has to find the right place (decidua) and implant. By day twelve, implantation has started to commence, eroding into the superficial layer of the decidua like a cancer. By day thirteen, it has to find a blood vessel, it has to establish what we call haemo-choridnal contact. So now it makes contact with maternal blood for the first time to set up its osmotic situation. And that has all got to take place before day fourteen.

If you think of all that, it is a constant wonder that it ever actually works. It's just an amazing event, so it's not surprising that 65 to 80 per cent of all conceptions die before a woman misses her period. It is not surprising that between 15 and 20 per cent of detected pregnancies are lost in early pregnancy. And that is why only 2.5 per cent of babies are born abnormal. Because, in our species, the selection process is done at the start.

～❡～

This is how Dr Steigrad explains the conception process, but most clinics have preliminary lectures, so specialists will explain this, and the proposed treatments, in their own way.

The Things That Can Go Wrong with Women

This is a brief summary of some of the most common conditions that affect women when they cannot conceive. Patients must, however, seek authoritative advice from a fertility specialist or clinic to determine their individual conditions.

There are many variations on conditions, and fertility specialists approach them in different ways. You must trust the doctor you have chosen, or find one you do trust.

Another thing all fertility specialists seem to agree on is the element of chance in fertility. Most of them will tell you that some people conceive with little medical chance of success, while others with seemingly nothing wrong cannot conceive. Within these unsatisfactory parameters, the following are some of the conception inhibitors.

Failure to ovulate

Without an egg, there can be no baby. This is why doctors usually suggest temperature charts in the initial phases to give them some indication of whether ovulation has taken place. A rise in temperature in the second half of the cycle indicates that it has done. Ovulation problems can be caused by an inadequate production of the hormones producing ovulation, or an imbalance in these hormones. In very severe cases, premature menopause may be diagnosed.

A hormone assay (analysis) will probably be suggested by the fertility specialist. This involves blood tests at intervals throughout a cycle. These will test the hormones involved in the process of ovulation — follicle stimulating hormone (FSH), luteinizing hormone (LH), oestrogen and progesterone. Also, another pituitary hormone, prolactin, usually produced by women when breastfeeding, will be tested, as this can interfere with normal secretion of FSH. Thyroid disorders have also been found to affect fertility adversely.

The measurement of these hormones, interpreted by an expert, can suggest the next stage in your fertility treatment.

Premature menopause or premature ovarian failure

If a woman ceases to have periods and begins to experience menopausal symptoms under the age of 40, she is diagnosed as having premature ovarian failure. Sometimes her periods stop after a period of lengthening cycles; sometimes they stop abruptly.

The ovaries stop producing the hormone oestrogen, so the typical menopausal symptoms of hot flushes, mood changes and vaginal dryness can commence. As the ovaries stop producing eggs, there is little chance of conception. There isn't always an explanation for this condition; sometimes it runs in families.

Some women can have a long period where ovaries are slowing down and ovulation may occur from time to time. This is called *resistant ovarian syndrome*, where the ovaries are resistant to the FSH and LH released.

These hormones are very high at menopause, as they are trying to encourage the ovaries to work. Elevated levels of these hormones indicate premature ovarian failure. Other hormones are usually checked at the same time to confirm the diagnosis.

Unfortunately, if premature ovarian failure is diagnosed, little can be done except for using donated eggs and IVF, after the doctors have created a hormone drug-induced cycle for you.

Tubal problems

This is one of the most common causes of infertility, and one which produced a diagnosis of sterility in the days before IVF.

The tubes must be open and move freely to collect the egg and also the minuscule interior passage must be undamaged, for the passage of the egg is dependent on the action of cells lining the tube and the muscular contractions of the tubes themselves. The interior of the tubes is covered with tiny hairs which beat together to push the ovum, sperm and embryo along. With the use of a falloposcopy, it is now possible to study the interior of the tube.

The use of intra-uterine devices for contraception is associated with infection and tubal blockage, and also the common use of the Pill as a contraceptive device — rather than a barrier method such as a condom — may have increased the risk of sexually transmitted diseases.

Pelvic inflammatory disease (PID) is a major health problem. It is usually accompanied by period-type pain, pain at intercourse, discharge, fever and frequent or painful urination. Any of these symptoms should be dealt with immediately, as the long-term effect on fertility can be profound. It is now much more widely publicised, and both patients and doctors are more aware of the need for swift diagnostic tests and treatment.

Endometriosis

It is still not known precisely how endometriosis develops, but it is a condition where the tissue that usually lines the uterus (the endometrium) grows in locations outside the uterus. The most popular theory about its cause is retrograde menstruation, where the menstrual fluid flows back into the pelvis via the Fallopian tubes.

This fluid contains blood and living tissue from the uterine lining, and somehow these fragments of tissue implant themselves on other organs and begin to grow and function. This means, they begin to respond to the menstrual hormones, and they break down and bleed in the same way as the endometrium itself, at period time. The blood cannot escape, so it bleeds onto the surrounding organs and tissues, causing irritation, which leads to scarring and sometimes adhesions between the organs.

Strong period pain is the most common symptom, but symptoms range from debilitating pain to almost no symptoms at all.

Polycystic ovarian syndrome

This is another common problem for couples having trouble conceiving. Polycystic literally means 'many cysts'. The cysts should really be termed follicles, however, as they are not indicators of some sinister disease, but are vital to the reproductive process, as follicles contain the eggs. In sufferers of this condition, ovaries are somewhat larger than average and contain about twice as many follicles as usual. About one in five women have this condition and only a small proportion will have fertility problems.

No one knows why a woman with polycystic ovaries goes on to develop polycystic ovarian syndrome and subfertility. The typical features of this syndrome combine disturbed or irregular menstruation with some degree of unwanted body hair. Excess hair does not appear with all patients.

About a third of women with this syndrome are overweight, indicating women with this condition may have a slightly different metabolism. Weight reduction can sometimes improve fertility. Blood tests are taken for women suspected of having this problem as most have evidence of a hormone imbalance, which may be a factor in ovulation problems.

Fortunately most women will be able to become pregnant by treatment with follicle stimulating hormone (FSH). Clomiphene (Clomid or Serophone) is usually the first treatment offered. This is usually given in tablet form and works by stimulating the body's own supply of FSH from the pituitary gland. It is usually prescribed for five days a few days after the start of the period. This is successful in about three-quarters of patients. For the other 25 per cent, FSH is usually given by injection, but supervised under specialist care to avoid overstimulating the ovary. As stated earlier, a calorie-controlled diet is important to overweight patients as response to drug therapy has been found to be better in women of normal weight.

Mucus hostility

Many patients claim that mucus hostility is blamed when nothing else can be found. The idea of having a hostile army of organisms around your cervix beating off the intruding sperm also has its funny side.

This diagnosis is reached after a post-coital test, where the couple make love at a time close to ovulation when the woman's mucus should be slippery and receptive, and the movement and survival of sperm in this mucus, taken from a sample a bit like a Pap smear test, is analysed, within a given time from intercourse occurring. Doctors have been disputing the effectiveness of this test and diagnosis since it was first performed in the 1860s. It does prove that intercourse has taken place in the correct way. However, anything further is dependent on the timing of ovulation. Rather than leaving it to the couple to determine approximately when ovulation is due, it is important to combine this test with clinical hormonal tests ensuring that the timing was correct. 'Hostile' mucus may sometimes just be mucus produced at slightly the wrong time, when looser estimates of ovulation are used.

A more sophisticated test is called the Kremer test or sperm-cervical mucus contact test, where cervical mucus at ovulation is placed into a long tube, the partner's sperm is placed in a small reservoir, and the glass tube is placed into this reservoir. Then the sperm movement and activity can be studied under the microscope. With this test, both sperm and mucus can be assessed. The mucus can also be tested with donor sperm, and the husband with donor mucus, to establish which, if any, are at fault. This test is also used to test males for antisperm antibodies (see later in the chapter).

Fibroids

Fibroids are solid, benign growths that appear on the outside, inside or within the wall of the uterus. About 30 per cent of all women will develop fibroids by the time they are 35 years old. The cause is unknown, but they are related to oestrogen production. When you are pregnant or taking hormones, fibroids often grow more quickly.

Again, there is dispute about the seriousness of fibroids in relation to fertility treatment. Many fibroids are small and on the outside wall of the uterus and cause no symptoms. However, as they usually grow during pregnancy, they can bulge inwards into the uterus and affect the foetal position or the placenta.

I had two major fibroids the size of tennis balls and a baby weighing more than 4 kilograms in my uterus at the end of my pregnancy. The only side-effect was that one fibroid was close to the cervix, so it couldn't dilate properly and I had to have a caesarean-section birth. The other negative side was that they hurt excruciatingly as I breastfed my son and the womb tried to contract. And his looks were not great for the first month, as he had pushed his head down beside the fibroid to the cervix, so his head was a bit lop-sided!

Some doctors believe fibroids within the uterus can prevent the implantation of the embryo, rather like an intra-uterine device. Your doctor will advise you of the seriousness of your fibroids, their location and what should be done about them, if anything. The operation to remove them is called a *myomectomy* and can be done by hysteroscopy (a tubelike fibre-optic scope, inserted through the vagina), by laparoscopy (a fine instrument inserted through a tiny incision near the belly button) or by an open operation. This will depend on their size and where they are growing. Hormone therapy may be given before the operation to reduce their size. Very often though, they do grow back again.

Recurrent miscarriage

The loss of a much-awaited pregnancy is one of the most tragic scenarios a couple can face. But to have this loss repeated several times is almost unendurable, one made more so by the lack of a tangible reason for the loss. The doctors can usually only quote statistics and hope for better luck next time. There are *four main causes* for early (in the first three months) miscarriages:

- **genetic problems**, where for some reason the fertilised egg doesn't divide as it must to further the development of the foetus. Some women actually have something called a *chemical pregnancy*, where they are not even aware they are pregnant and miscarry before it is detected. Egg age can be a factor in these early pregnancy losses, where the foetus may otherwise have been abnormal. If there is a family history of genetic disorders, couples may seek genetic counselling.
- **anatomical problems**, caused by some abnormality in the woman's tubes or uterus may interrupt a pregnancy. Damaged Fallopian tubes can lead to a tubal pregnancy, where the fertilised egg attaches itself to the interior of the tube, not the uterus, and begins to grow there. Immediate surgery is required to remove this as it will soon

outgrow the tube and rupture it. Doctors are now using a drug to dissolve a tubal pregnancy, thus perhaps saving the affected tube, and not requiring surgery. This can only be used very early in the development of a tubal pregnancy.

- **hormonal imbalances**, which are suspected if a woman has only a short number of days after she has ovulated and before her period arrives. In a normal ovulation, this luteal phase is a fairly standard time of between 11 and 17 days. This marks the time where the corpus luteum, the residual endocrine structure in the follicle where the egg ruptured, produces progesterone to enrich the lining of the womb for implantation. The corpus luteum supports the pregnancy in the first 8–10 weeks, creating nourishment for the developing foetus, until the placenta is established and can take over. A pathologist can measure the maturity of the endometrium or womb lining, and if it is insufficient, it means the hormones are not functioning properly.

    Progesterone levels may also be measured and progesterone injections or suppositories given to sustain the pregnancy if the levels are found to be low.

- **unknown causes** — this frustrating diagnosis encompasses the large majority or early pregnancy failures. However, as medical science progresses, more causes are being identified. As doctors work with IVF techniques, they are learning about early foetal development and what can go wrong.

Things That Can Go Wrong with Men

Unlike a woman, who is born with all the eggs she will ever have, a man's testicles produce millions of new sperm every day, starting at puberty and continuing into old age. Unfortunately, in most cases of subfertility in men, causes are not easily identified.

Sperm take about 75 days to develop and mature in the testicles. They move then from a duct next to the testicle, constantly undergoing changes, into the vas deferens, which is a thicker tube, able to be felt in the groin region of men. Most of the sperm are stored in a little pocket at the end of the vas deferens. In ejaculation, glandular secretions and muscular contractions combine to move the semen through the penis. Along the way, the semen is joined by other fluids so the sperm make up only a small proportion of the ejaculate. Because the urethra, the main tube in the penis, also carries the urine, at ejaculation, a valve closes so sperm cannot enter the bladder. After the semen is ejaculated, it forms a thick, gluey substance, which liquefies again in 5 to 20 minutes.

When the sperm are ejaculated into the vagina, they must be good swimmers and dash up the uterus and into the tubes. This property is known as *motility*. Sperm continues maturing as it swims and this process is the capacitation mentioned in Dr Steigrad's lecture. This is necessary so that the sperm are capable of penetrating the egg surface. Estimates vary on how long sperm can live in the woman's reproductive tract, but it is thought to be about 48 hours.

A semen analysis is usually one of the first tests called for. This determines if the ejaculate actually contains sperm, how they look (morphology) and how well they swim (motility). *Azoospermia* means there is no sperm present at all and *oligospermia* means that there are only small numbers of sperm there. A doctor will usually examine the man for abnormalities in the testicles and penis, and hormone levels can be tested from a blood sample. Chapter 9, on artificial insemination, deals more fully with the physical and emotional implications of a poor sperm count.

Varicoceles

A *varicocele* is a kind of varicose vein in the scrotum. The doctor can usually feel this during a manual examination. Experts don't know why this affects sperm quality, but suspect it inhibits blood flow, causing the temperature of the scrotum to rise. Surgery can correct this and make blood flow normal, and improve fertility.

Blockages

Blockages in the reproductive tract can make men who are producing good sperm infertile. Testicular biopsy can check whether blockages exist and the doctor can determine whether they can be corrected.

Retrograde ejaculation

Retrograde ejaculation can occur if the valve at the opening of the bladder is faulty and sperm are escaping into the urinary tract.

Absence of the vas deferens

In a very rare number of men, the vas deferens is absent due to a birth defect. This is only present in about 2 per cent of males, but a blockage of the vas deferens is the cause about 20 to 30 per cent of obstructions.

Endocrine disorders

Abnormalities in the endocrine gland system account for about 20 per cent of infertility in men — in general, abnormalities in the testicle, hypothalamus or pituitary. So measuring male hormone levels can help doctors identify what is causing the problem, and if medication is appropriate. The hormones LH, FSH and testosterone are important at the start of sperm production.

Klinefelter's syndrome

Klinefelter's syndrome is a genetic anomaly in which the chromosomal numbers are abnormal. Men with this syndrome produce no sperm. These men are likely to be tall with little facial or body hair, and very small, inactive testes. Sexual potency is present, but sperm are entirely absent.

Antibodies

Antibodies can impair fertility for men and women. Just as the body's immune system produces antibodies to fight off bacteria, for some reason, the immune systems of some people recognise sperm as an intruder and attack them.

The percentages of this problem are higher in men whose infertility is due to a block allowing sperm to build up in the body. This problem is common in about 60 per cent of men who have undergone a vasectomy. This is one reason successful reversal of vasectomies is hard — especially when the vasectomy was performed more than three years before the attempted reversal.

Undescended testes

Undescended testes are usually diagnosed in early life, but doctors examining the male partner will check that both testicles have descended.

Infection

Mumps are probably the most common culprit causing irreversible damage to sperm production. Also, sexually transmitted diseases such as gonorrhea can cause blockages in the ducts.

Chemotherapy

Chemotherapy usually stops sperm production, but it may resume after therapy has been stopped. Doctors will advise you on how long you should wait between treatment and trying for a family. Often, cancer patients are advised to freeze some undamaged sperm before treatment begins, for use later.

Drugs

Some drugs may affect sperm production. Alcohol, tranquillisers and narcotics all depress the production of sperm. They may also depress the libido.

Unexplained Infertility

This frustrating non-diagnosis greets couples who have, after extensive tests, been found to have no abnormalities, but who cannot conceive. It is also referred to as idiopathic infertility. For most couples, it is easier if a problem is actually uncovered, which can then be attacked or treated. Unfortunately, for people facing unexplained infertility, there are no ready answers.

In a social sense, this makes them the target of all those fertile do-gooders who trot out the cliches about going on holiday, or suggest that in some way they aren't doing IT correctly. Sometimes doctors offer treatments hoping to overcome the unknown causes.

Hormone treatments may be suggested. Intra-uterine insemination with the partner's sperm may be suggested. GIFT treatment may be suggested, where the eggs are stimulated and collected and then replaced into the Fallopian tube with the partner's sperm. Doctors may then suggest IVF.

If these treatments are unsuccessful, however, a couple can only hope that one day a pregnancy will happen or they can try to make a life without children, or with adopted or foster children.

Chapter 4
Call for Help

Definition: A couple is regarded as infertile when they have not conceived after 12 months of regular, unprotected sexual intercourse.
ACCESS Fact Sheet

~ e ~

'You have a right to consider yourself infertile whenever you begin to feel concerned about your failure to become pregnant.'
The New Our Bodies, Ourselves,
The Boston Women's Health Book Collective

Having spent so many years trying to avoid pregnancy, everyone is sure they will become pregnant the first month they have unprotected intercourse.

I still remember the chilling day when I was about 32 and my new (short-lived) gynaecologist told me that my intra-uterine device probably wouldn't need changing as the years of using these devices had probably made me sterile. It was the first time it had occurred to me that my fertility might have a time span. I decided there and then that he wasn't the doctor for me, and also that it might be a good idea, now that I was settled into a strong relationship and a good career, to let fate take a hand and not do anything about contraception.

Heading off on a trip to London and New York with my partner, it simply never occurred to me I wouldn't be pregnant by the time I got back to Sydney. Every month after that I was sure would be THE MONTH, although as both my partner and I had had pregnancies, I didn't worry for a couple of years. And if I did, I just assumed we were not timing things correctly — my cycle had a mind of its own, varying from 21 to 26 days. The anxiety did not set in for some time.

The months when I did think we'd timed everything to perfection, I did start running to the loo a lot to see if there was a trace of a period starting, then felt an inner glow if it hadn't. Inserting a tampon gives an even earlier indication of blood traces for the very impatient, like me. So why wasn't anything happening?

These selected comments from other couples reflect the same bewilderment:

'In hindsight, I believe we waited too long before seeking help from the specialists at a fertility clinic. We had always planned to have children and it was something we looked forward to, but [we] wanted to establish ourselves professionally, financially and personally before having a family. My approaching 30th birthday, after seven years of marriage, was the catalyst. I was not overly concerned when

we failed to conceive within the first few months of trying. I knew that after coming off the Pill it could take up to a year to conceive. Also, as I worked at night and we didn't spend as much time together as other couples, I thought perhaps we weren't having regular enough sex. Before going off the Pill, I approached my GP with the news that we were ready at last to start a family. She had previously asked me if we were ever planning to have children, suggesting that "nice people should have children". So I was sent off for a blood test to check my immunity to rubella, which was still current after the shots all 13-year-old girls receive. My doctor revealed that she was planning baby number three and suggested we have a little competition to see who would become pregnant first. When I failed to become pregnant within a year, I telephoned her office for an appointment, only to be told that she had given up work at the practice as she had just given birth,' recounted one woman, as yet unsuccessful in her treatment.

'After a few years of marriage we had a discussion one day about starting a family. I just said which day do you want to have a baby? Would you prefer a winter or summer baby? It doesn't work like that, does it?' one husband said.

'We just thought we'd have Joe's vasectomy reversed, and I'd be pregnant in no time,' a woman added.

'It was a second marriage for both of us,' said a British woman, 'and at first children were not on the agenda, even though I was 40 and my husband 42. I wanted a baby for about 12 to 18 months before talking to my husband about our failure to conceive. I read everything I could get my hands on and tried everything before I actually talked with my husband about my worries.'

Maybe because men are more matter-of-fact and fatalistic about their bodies and procreation, the prevailing attitude for them is often if it is meant to happen it will, if not, it won't. In contrast, women are so used to their monthly ebb and flow, literally, that they are attuned to the slightest variation. They rarely lose track of their cycles, particularly if they are trying to achieve a pregnancy, so the few days before their period is due and the few days after are spent in full focus. Breast tenderness, a spot on the chin, PMT or a delayed period are all reminders each month of failure to conceive.

No matter how loving or supportive our partners are, they just don't have the same physical or emotional awareness. The longer the time we spend trying to conceive without seeking help, the greater the build-up of tension and anxiety. By the time we actually see a fertility specialist or even our general practitioner, we have already built up multiple scenarios, usually apportioning blame for 'failure' to ourselves or to our partners.

Because no one knows how often is 'normal' for sexual intercourse, we all feel our sexuality is on trial when we go to the doctor to report our failure to conceive. It doesn't matter how sophisticated we think we are. Frequency of intercourse is one of the first questions the doctors ask. Except in one case:

I was a child-bride who grew up and my husband, considerably older, didn't really want biological children. I gathered up my courage and announced I wanted a baby. From that day on, he didn't make love to me. But he agreed to my going to have some tests, although he refused a semen test as he said there could be no question of something being wrong with him. I had a standard D&C (dilation and curettage), did some temperature charts and whatever else they did in those days, but no one ever asked me did we have sexual intercourse. We didn't any more. My husband wouldn't touch me. But I was too embarrassed to tell anyone.

Seeking Help

The first call for most of us is usually the general practitioner's surgery or the bookstore. I had bought the one volume in the bookstore on infertility and had been busily keeping temperature charts for some time. My chart looked normal, so my doctor and I deduced I was at least ovulating. I had the grim prediction of the unsympathetic gynaecologist in my brain telling me that my tubes would probably be blocked after all those years with an intra-uterine device, but I also knew that I had been aware of the dangers with an intra-uterine device (IUD) and meticulously had it changed on schedule every two years — or whenever the doctor advised me. I also knew that the redeeming feature of my charming gynaecologist, who had presumably been careless in inserting an IUD without a D&C when I was already in very early pregnancy (or maybe the pregnancy was in the tube still, to give him the benefit of the doubt), was that each time he changed my IUD he insisted on it being done in hospital under surgical conditions and he also prescribed two weeks of no intercourse, no tampons and antibiotics each time it was changed. So I did know every care had been taken to protect my fertility — and me — from infection, even though the use of IUD's was still controversial for those who hadn't had children.

From sharing other patients' experiences, I also feel that secondary infertility, such as ours, was puzzling, but marginally less traumatic than for those who had never had a pregnancy, male or female. Because you have experienced it, you don't have quite the sense of psychological barrenness as those who have never had a pregnancy.

My GP sent me off to see a new and wonderful gynaecologist to find out why nothing was happening. He referred us to a specialist fertility clinic. Most doctors ask you to do a few months of preliminary temperature charts—the least invasive way of telling if you are ovulating. A temperature rise in the second half of the cycle suggests that ovulation has taken place. When you are given temperature charts, you also have to mark the days you had intercourse. I wonder how many of us tell the truth? Isn't it always the way that at the critical moment when the temperature drops, one of you is sick, away on business or definitely not in the mood. I used to make my timid marks with a cross; I have a friend who made her marks by drawing little red hearts. Most of us add an extra few crosses or hearts, thinking the chart looks a bit sparse.

Sometimes, if a man or a woman is aware of a possible problem, he or she seeks help immediately without waiting the usual twelve months, like the following woman:

My case was a little different. My husband and I have been together for 15 years — since I was 15 and he was 17. We always knew we could have fertility problems because at 16 I was diagnosed as possibly having polycystic ovarian syndrome and after being discharged from hospital at 17, I was told we would probably need help to conceive and to let my doctor know as soon as we wanted to start a family.

We discussed it as soon as I was told, decided our days of planning a family were a long way off and we'd get on with the rest of our lives in the meantime. It was seven years later, having moved back to our home town that we decided we would throw away the Pill and try for a family.

It was about three months before we went to the doctor and, knowing what we did, they were very good and referred us directly to the hospital to begin the endless round of tests. Because this was in England, we had to wait about 12 months for tests, and after every test known was performed on me, including a laparoscopy and dye test, they finally did a test on my husband's semen. I think it was about two years down the line.

Others have had a range of experiences. The woman whose former GP had beaten her in the race to have a baby went to see the replacement doctor:

The new GP suggested temperature charts and mucus readings for the next few months. After about six months with no success, we approached her again. This time my husband was sent off for a semen analysis, the results of which were poor, but the GP didn't seem too concerned. She said 'One is all you need', the cliche we've since heard repeated so often.

She suggested we keep trying for another six months, which we did. My husband never felt comfortable with this new GP, believing she was too flippant suggesting things like try wearing boxer shorts. When still nothing happened, we were sent off to a fertility clinic.

When the fertility clinician opened our letter of referral and noted the sperm analysis, he proclaimed it would be difficult for us to conceive without assisted reproductive technology. He said: 'Some people say it takes only one sperm, but that is not the case.' My husband and I immediately cast each other a glance: it was the opposite to the information we had been given.

Some women report that it is standard practice in their region to be referred straight to a specialist fertility clinic after one year of trying to conceive. Another adds her experience:

I knew I would have difficulties as my husband was a Vietnam war veteran and had had a vasectomy as he was fearful of the birth defects which were occurring with fellow veterans. So we always knew we would have to use donor sperm. However, I went to one local doctor and explained our case and he refused me a referral to a fertility clinic because my husband is thirty years my senior and he said it wouldn't be fair on the child. I decided he wasn't the only local doctor I could see and that he had no right whatever to tell me whether I should or shouldn't have children. I found another doctor and he referred us straight away to the fertility clinic at our local hospital.

In Australia these days, patients are fairly lucky and there are not long waiting lists in most places. This is not the case in the United Kingdom, where even the preliminary tests have long waiting times, and this adds considerably to the stress. Many patients dip into their savings or borrow to speed up the process by using private care.

Because I was over 40, I was referred straight to a fertility specialist. We agreed to have my tests done privately for speed, as in England the waiting lists are long. My husband's semen analysis came back through our local doctor. When we went for the results, she was terribly nervous and apologetic. She said she had had very little sleep as she had two patients she had to give bad news to. One was dying of cancer. The other was us — my husband was azoospermic. My husband reacted very calmly, I think he may have suspected.

Australia may not have the pressing population of other countries such as the United Kingdom, but there are other obstacles to overcome. Distance is one of them. Now clinics in some major centres have developed satellite clinics to help couples receive expert care in rural areas. The local doctors do preliminary testing before patients arrive in the larger centre for treatment. Like the following case:

In our area of Northern Queensland, the procedure is that the semen analysis and laparoscopies are done locally before you are referred to the major clinic. All females must have a laparoscopy and all males a semen analysis, and then the clinic has a fair idea what they are dealing with.

The Specialists

Dr Stephen Steigrad suggests that if general practitioners could be educated more in the latest procedures of assisted fertility, they could short-circuit some of the duplication of testing now done. He stated that the laboratories testing semen samples can vary a lot, and if your own doctor orders this test, he or she should send it to a specialist laboratory for analysis, avoiding the duplication when the couple arrive at the fertility clinic if the analysis is substandard.

He also believes couples should be sent directly to fertility specialists, rather than to a more general gynaecologist/obstetrician. He said:

I don't believe that the generalist obstetrician/gynaecologist is the ideal person to start investigations for infertility because he or she may be distracted by the pressures of other things within the practice. If you go to someone who is making a speciality of infertility, they are probably in a better position to investigate patients. It doesn't always mean they'll be very good; there may be patient–doctor failure of interaction and the patient should be prepared to change doctor. But at least they should be abreast of the latest treatments. Doctors can make patients feel very vulnerable. Patients must realise that they can always ask for a second opinion if they have any worries or anxieties.'

Dr Steigrad was my own second opinion. The first clinic I was referred to seemed fine, but I didn't like the doctor. I'm sure clinically he was good, but the way he told me about my partner's semen analysis, plus his brusque manner and abrupt way of telling me what we should do next — or not — made me think we would never have a good patient–doctor rapport. I was vulnerable and felt I needed someone a bit more human. Without really telling me what GIFT was, he said it was an option for us, then went on to tell me how many multiple pregnancies they'd had that year — quads, triplets and twins. This was before doctors had put a self-limitation on the number of eggs or embryos replaced. As an aunt of a pair of very difficult twins, I knew my partner and I could probably cope with twins (just), but quads or triplets, I felt I could be on my own.

Also, in my 12 years of working on the *Australian Women's Weekly*, we had had several stories revealing the hardships of multiple births — the side-effects of very premature birth for the babies and the marital kickback of dealing with these difficulties. One at around that time sticks in my mind, the story of a family of premature quintuplets, most of whom ended up blind and with cerebral palsy from their premature births. Divorce followed not many years later, from the pressure of raising them.

I went back to my usual gynaecologist and told him my fears and he said he'd refer me to his colleague within the hospital, Dr Steigrad. Now his bedside manner is not perfect — he also has a tendency to be brusque — but he was direct and no-nonsense, and I trusted him, the hospital and my gynaecologist's recommendation. That trust is critical. Some doctors inspire it, others don't, as the following experiences reveal:

I had never consulted a medical specialist and had never had a male doctor conduct any personal examinations before. But our clinician is a real gem and from the first meeting with him I have always felt very comfortable. My husband gets on well with him. Other women have told me that their specialists, because of the nature of their work, don't relate very well to the husbands. So I feel very fortunate. I think it is just as important for the male partner to feel comfortable with the couple's fertility specialist. While waiting in the mornings a lot of merriment is heard as he consults couples in his office. He has a marvellous sense of humour; I believe he can read his patients to know how far his brand of humour can be received. On one occasion, while waiting for an embryo transfer, strapped in stirrups with legs almost touching the ceiling and feeling most uncomfortable, my clinician, ready to carry out the transfer, pulled back the sheet and declared, 'Now I recognise her.' Everyone, including the nurses, burst into laughter and I relaxed. But I understand his brand of humour would not be appreciated by everyone.

Not all doctors strike the right note between formality and informality. But couples in Australia are at least fortunate that most doctors no longer have a God complex and do try to put you at ease in these emotional and often uncomfortable situations. Some, obviously, do it better than others:

'Male doctors always seem to want to talk to the males. They're always sharing a joke and I think, what about me? My husband thinks our specialist is a good doctor and a good joker. One really positive thing though, he never, ever makes you feel uncomfortable. When he had to be serious he could be serious.'

Her husband comments: 'I think he was serious when he was talking about his putting order.'

'One examination with my doctor, he left me lying naked on the couch for about 20 minutes while he took a personal phone call,' said a Melbourne patient. 'It was freezing. He came in as if nothing had happened. When he examined me he said the same old, usual thing, "Now I recognise you" when he lifted the sheet — I think that must be the standard gynaecologist joke.'

'My GP gave me an open-ended referral to the fertility clinic, and I asked how long do you think I'm going to go for, this is ridiculous,' said another woman.

Small towns and lack of choice also have their drawbacks:

I had a history of no periods, so I knew there could be a problem. We lived in a small country town and the choice of specialists was not great. One of the local doctors had a particularly bad attitude and had no concept of the difficult emotional state we were in. While we were struggling to remember it was our problem, not just mine, he would in effect try and form a boys' club with my husband.

For example, when we visited him to find out the results of my husband's sperm test, he got up from the chair, shook my husband's hand and said, 'We have no worries with you, you could populate the whole of the town with your results.' On another occasion, just after this doctor had performed a D&C on me, I asked

YOUR RIGHTS

ACCESS, Australia's national fertility support group, produces a fact sheet entitled *How To Get the Best out of Your Health Professional*. Under the section called 'Your rights', it states:

1. You have the right to be treated in a humane manner with care, consideration and dignity.
2. You should be given a clear, concise explanation in non-medical terms of your problem.
3. You should be given a clear, concise explanation of any treatment or investigation, including whether such treatment is of an experimental nature.
4. You have the right to have your partner in the consulting room with you.
5. You are entitled to refuse: an examination, a particular treatment or operation.
6. You have the right to ask for a second opinion, i.e. to see another doctor. Ask the specialist you are seeing or ask your general practitioner to refer you to another specialist.
7. You have the right to see your medical file, but you can't take it away. You can nominate a doctor (usually your GP) to obtain all your medical records and to inform you of what they contain. [NB In France, I was surprised and pleased to find that the patient was trusted to keep their own obstetrics file — so practical in case you were away somewhere and had an emergency. Also, copies of all tests are sent to the patient as well as the doctor, so the Anglo-Saxon passion for secrecy *from* the patient doesn't exist.]

By Dr Sue Craig © ACCESS, reprinted with permission.

my husband to ask him how long I could expect to bleed after the operation. This was in the recovery room. The doctor looked at me and turned to my husband and said, 'She'll be good for it by Monday night.'

I immediately asked my local doctor for a referral back to my former doctor in Sydney. Even though it was a 200-mile round trip, I would rather do that than stay with this local so-called professional. My Sydney doctor was much more in tune with the fact that this was a serious issue for both of us as people and as a married couple.

Some of the stress disappears when you have found the specialist or clinic with whom or with which you feel comfortable. Whereas before you may have felt you had no chance of conceiving, now you are beginning an exciting journey that you hope will culminate in a baby.

Specialists everywhere begin by wanting a clear picture of your current reproductive health. For the male, they need a semen analysis done by a recognised laboratory.

YOUR RESPONSIBILITIES

1. Be assertive. Ask, insist, tell, confront, book, change, refuse, persist, understand and question.
2. Be well informed. Join a self-help group, read literature.
3. Join a private health fund. This enables choice of specialist and treatment; allays costs in the long term.
4. Keep your own records of all tests, results and treatments.
5. Make a list of questions before your appointment, and write down the answers. If you wish to tape the interview, ask for permission.
6. Book a long appointment if you feel you need more time with the doctor.
7. Inform the doctor or his receptionist if you are unable to attend a consultation.
8. Take your partner with you to the doctor if you both wish to be involved. It can be mutually supportive.
9. Defer any treatment if you are unsure about it.
10. Have reasonable expectations about your health professional. Understand he/she may be tired, rushed or unwell.
11. If you cannot communicate with your doctor, it is in your interest to find someone with whom you can talk.
12. If you are dissatisfied with your treatment, try and discuss this with the doctor.
13. If you need to speak with the doctor, ring the surgery, leave your name, phone number and message, rather than interrupt him/her during consultations.
14. If you have unexplained infertility and all investigations and treatments have been tried, you may like to return to your doctor every two years to check on new developments in infertility treatment that may help you.

By Dr Sue Craig © ACCESS, reprinted with permission

For the female, some doctors require temperature charts to get a regular picture of the woman's monthly cycles, others take a progesterone test in what would be the post-ovulation (luteal) phase of the cycle. In a normal cycle, this is around day 21 to day 25. If the progesterone has reached a required level, they can deduce that ovulation has taken place.

The specialist also needs to establish that the woman's Fallopian tubes, used to transport the egg from the ovary to the uterus, are clear and healthy for the sperm and egg to travel through, meet and combine. This is established by a test where dye is fed into the uterus via a small tube through the cervix and forced through the uterus into the tubes. If it disperses through the end of the tubes, all is well. This is called a hystersalpingogram or HSG, and can be done without anaesthetic or under anaesthetic at the same time as the laparoscopy. The condition of the interior walls of the tubes must also be good as they perform a sweeping function for both sperm and egg.

Most specialists will also want to perform a laparoscopy, done under anaesthetic, to check the internal organs. A small camera is inserted via a tube into the stomach through a tiny cut near the navel. The stomach is inflated with gas so the doctor can have a clear picture of all the organs. Adhesions, thin threads which may hamper free movement of the ovaries or tubes, and endometriosis, where the endometrium (womb lining) is shed via the tubes into the stomach cavity instead of into the menstrual flow, can be picked up this way.

They may also ask you to undergo a post-coital test at ovulation time, where you make love and then go off to the lab for a test like a smear test, to check the quality of the woman's mucus and its interaction with her partner's sperm.

These are the basic tests needed to give the specialist a clear picture of your chances of conceiving. Most fertility specialists will insist on these basic tests so they can go forward with you to plan your treatment. But you must also be aware of the tests you should have and insist you have them.

On some occasions, patients have had one partner showing an obvious problem, like a poor sperm count or poor ovulation, and the treatment has been centred on that partner for some time before the other partner is thoroughly tested. Several stressful months or even years later, when a test is finally done on the other partner, a more major problem may be found with that person. So part of your assertion with your doctor must be, if he or she doesn't suggest it, that you both have these basic tests:

- semen analysis at a specialist laboratory
- post-coital test
- laparoscopy
- test for tubal viability
- temperature charts or progesterone test to check for ovulation.

This avoids scenarios such as the British woman with polycystic ovarian syndrome who had two years of intensive testing before someone decided to test her husband. As she said: 'I went through two years of tests before they did anything with my husband. It was only then they did a sperm test and found my husband was producing no sperm whatsoever, and my problem was unimportant by comparison.'

A patient in Melbourne, Australia, had a similar problem in reverse:

My husband had had testicular cancer and had one testicle removed and chemotherapy, so we knew we had to wait five years before even trying for a family. When the cancer specialist had a semen analysis done, he told us that the count was low, but there certainly were some good sperm there. He referred us to an infertility specialist. The doctor told us he wanted to do a routine laparoscopy on me.

I thought to myself and said to my husband outside the surgery, 'Don't be stupid, there's nothing wrong with me. We all know it's you.' (This was said lovingly). I had my laparoscopy, D&C and dye test and was shocked to learn I had very bad adhesions around my tubes.

I was told in a post-operative daze that both my tubes were blocked. The professor rang me a few days later to make sure I'd understood. I was quite shocked, but my husband and I joked that at least we were both duds, neither of us could blame the other.

Another woman cites a similar case:

Because of sperm problems following my husband's vasectomy reversal, the clinic automatically assumed there was nothing wrong with me. We've been through three ICSI treatments and they've never tested me. I could be growing mushrooms in there. Every time I ask them they say, 'But it is your husband who has the problem.'

Her friend adds: 'I've had the reverse. When they told me I had to have a laparoscopy, I told them it was my husband with the problem, but they said I had to have a laparoscopy, too. It is so important to have a total picture of both partners.'

Summing up

I think they should teach about infertility in schools the same way they teach about contraception and anorexia and all the other health issues, so we are aware of it. We are all now trying to have children in our late 20s and 30s. If we knew about potential problems in our teens, we wouldn't have wasted time. The problems I had as a 15-year-old were not treated. They just prescribed the Pill in those days for anyone with problem periods. Then when you do decide you want a family, it is too late. You may have ten or more years of damage done.

If I'd been told at 15 or 16. 'Don't muck around, don't put it off,' at least I would have had a choice. When you do find out you have a problem, it often leaves you very little time to fix it. I also suggest if you think you've got a problem like this to tell the doctors you've been trying for two or three years so they do something immediately. If you have to wait to hit that magic 12 months of trying so you are an officially infertile person, you've wasted even more time.

Professor Carl Wood, Australia's pioneer of in vitro fertilisation (IVF), has a different perspective:

Education should probably precede the teenage years. Some education programs in late primary school have been more effective than waiting till the teenage years. This may be because if you wait till puberty, emotional factors and sexual feeling make acceptance of advice more difficult. There is now good evidence that the Pill does reduce the risk of recurrence of endometriosis by 50 per cent. Using the Pill may delay the onset of symptoms, but if it does so it is most likely to have delayed the progression of the disease as the symptoms are very dependent on the active process of the disease. Diseases such as endometriosis and fibroids are dependent on the number of periods a woman has. In our grandmothers' day, most women only had about 30 to 50 periods in their whole life, whereas today they may have 3000–4000 periods. The Pill can be used to reduce the amount of menstrual loss and also produce periods every two or three months, so this may have an important preventative role in these diseases.

I wish I had realised that the age of the maternal egg played such a huge role in fertility. Even when I started research for this book, I thought the negative talk about 'elderly primigravidas' was some kind of ageist plot with doctors playing the role of social scientist and preferring younger mothers because they were more socially acceptable or more convenient.

My interview with Dr Steigrad and subsequent doctors soon made me face the reality. Then I felt guilty that as a magazine editor and a member of the media for twenty-five years I had not known this and publicised it in some way. The media of the 1980s and early 1990s was too busy publicising the joys of motherhood for actresses and Italian grandmothers way into their 40s and sometimes later.

We were gravely at fault, as we peddled the idea of eternal youth. It suited us, the baby-boomers, busily following our professions, to think we could have babies on cue, as well as postpone them till it was convenient. We thought, erroneously, that youthfulness/fitness equals fertility/potency.

Perhaps the medical profession didn't communicate strictly enough with medical journalists. They didn't get the message across that we were playing a dangerous game delaying our offspring until it was often too late.

I'm grateful that it wasn't quite too late for me, but I have many friends and colleagues who weren't so lucky, as we tried to change the world and prove we could have it all.

Chapter 5
Testing Times

'I can cope with all the tests, I can cope with anything
except the stream of cliches.'
... the silent cry of every patient

HELPFUL HANNAH SAYS YOU'LL GET PREGNANT FOR SURE IF YOU JUST ...

- adopt a child
- go on holiday
- give up your job
- change your job
- eat your parsley
- try acupuncture
- lose your job
- move house
- break a leg
- sleep to the north–south, not the east–west
- increase your overdraft
- get drunk
- change your partner
- get very drunk
- file for divorce
- stop thinking about it and relax
- don't eat your parsley
- eat only foods starting with the letter 'c'
- trade in your sensible sedan for a Suzuki hatch
- keep no more than two of each utensil in your kitchen drawer
- elevate your bed

Reprinted from the *Friends of the Queensland Fertility Group* Newsletter, with a grateful 'Amen' from all patients who have had to suffer the well-meaning advice of friends, 'experts', mothers and mothers-in-law.

I was one of the lucky ones. I escaped the usual cliches. I simply didn't tell anyone how much I wanted a baby. Most friends and family thought we had such an enviable way of life, we had chosen careers and lifestyle over babies.

The really helpful opinion I received was from my businesswoman friend, who asked me very bluntly why I thought I should be able to 'have it all'—great but stressful work, glamorous lifestyle, travel ... and a baby. I don't think it directly affected my pregnancy, but it rang around in my head for many months and probably contributed to my decision to leave work when our son was born. I asked my doctor if stress played a role in infertility or miscarriage, and he said no one was sure for women, but it certainly affected the sperm counts of men.

My instincts told me that it couldn't really help things. The stress of running a magazine in a competitive market within a large, competitive organisation is fairly unrelenting. Also, every time work was at its most hassled, the part of my body that seemed to react was my lower abdomen, which went into a tight spasm. So I didn't think this could be entirely helpful to the luscious blood flow and warm receptive uterus I hoped would make a nice home for my prospective baby. Between the cliches and the self-diagnosis we all put ourselves through, however, there is only one place to truly start: we must all undergo tests — some simple, some more invasive.

Temperature Charts

Most doctors ask for a few months of temperature charts, just to get an idea of the length of your cycles, and see if it is probable that you are ovulating — seen by a dip around the middle of the cycle in a standard monthly chart, and a slightly raised temperature in the last 14 days of the cycle.

Patients have a love/hate relationship with the thermometer. In the investigative stage of things, I didn't mind the thermometer. It was fairly simple to get into the habit of taking my temperature each morning before I got up — the cat simply had to scream his Siamese call and *wait* for his breakfast. As my chart was pretty normal, it was quite reassuring that at least something was working.

Others had different ideas about this. One rural patient said:

I hated the thermometer. It interfered with our sex life and first thing in the morning I couldn't read it accurately or we would fall back to sleep and forget how long it was supposed to be used for. Then I bought a digital one that beeped and we made jokes about it being our alarm clock.

My doctor in Sydney used to fax up the fertility chart and the only access I had to a fax at the time was at work. So I used to hover over the fax (it was very slow, owing to all the grid lines) terrified that someone would come over and see what I was doing, or worse, the doctor might fax back and someone else would collect the fax.

Some had a more flippant reaction:

'I hated the thermometer, it was a pain in the backside,' said one woman. 'Well, you were putting it in the wrong place,' a male friend comments.

'They break every couple of weeks,' said one husband. Another responded, 'Well, you are not supposed to throw them on the ground.'

'It was hard for me — I wear contact lenses, so my husband had to read it.'

A different perspective: 'I got quite fond of it, but didn't use it after the fertility treatment really began.'

Most people found it reminded them daily of their quest for a child and took the spontaneity out of their sex lives: 'I didn't hate the thermometer so much; I hated the idea of having sex at this particular time on this particular day, it took all the fun out of it.'

Dr Steigrad explained the reason many clinics and doctors use them, although they are aware they are not a totally accurate guide to ovulation.

> There are a lot of arguments about basal temperature charts. They're not all that accurate. But we find they are very helpful because they provide a visual record whereby we can see what is going on and so can the patient. We can then explain what is happening to the patient clearly.
>
> I acknowledge it is a nuisance, it is a daily reminder of one's infertility, but it is valuable to us. We can say to the patient, 'this happened at this point and that's when your temperature went up,' and it makes a big difference. Also, it is something the patient can do to contribute to their treatment.
>
> We are also using home ovulation kits so patients can test themselves, so they are actually tracking their own cycles and ovulations at home. We realise it is convenient as they don't have to travel to the clinic for daily blood tests, but it may be more significant than that in that it involves the patient in her own management, and that is very positive.

Semen Analysis or Sperm Count

Several couples recount their experiences of collecting their semen sample. 'Well, I used to work in a lab, so I said to my husband this is what you've got to do, put it in a jar and I'll take it in. I used to look at them and do the counts.'

'I just basically gave my husband the jar,' said another, 'and he did it all by himself and put it in a jar and delivered it. He's kind of quiet and modest, so I didn't ask many questions. I offered assistance, but he said he didn't need it.'

Getting the sample to the laboratory within the right time frame is also a logistics exercise, as the following woman tells:

> The first time we had a sperm test, my husband refused to drive the sample to the clinic. I was told to drive with the specimen jar sitting between my legs. When I arrived at the pathology clinic, a nasty woman loudly questioned my marital status in front of a full waiting room (in a small country town) and the method of collection. I was very tempted to tell her oral and ask for a glass of water. However, with a flaming red face, I muttered the right response and feeling very embarrassed fled as quickly as possible after filling in the forms.

A sense of humour helps in most of these situations. 'It was always someone else's misfortune that seemed funny,' said one man. 'A friend lived too far away from the clinic to meet the time schedule, so he had to go to a building site where he was CEO and find some peace and quiet there. This poor bloke was desperate, searching for a quiet place.'

Others are very private in their collection method:

They sent me home with a bottle for my husband to do his sperm test. Which wasn't very easy. Basically we had to start to make love and then he had to rush off to the bathroom to finish it off, so to speak. Which wasn't very nice, but it was the only way we could complete the test.

The Post-Coital Test

This is where you really have to perform on demand, and seems to be, for many patients, the test requiring the most logistical planning. If your job is near your home which in turn is near the clinic, as mine were, it is fairly easy.

However, because the idea of this test is to see how well the mucus and sperm interact (the mucus must be like egg white, thin and slippery to activate and help the sperm in its journey through the uterus and up the tube), it is essential to do the test close to ovulation time, when this kind of mucus is produced. It is also important to get to the laboratory for the test to be taken within the number of hours your doctor requires.

And all this has to happen within the times the lab you are using is actually open. Not easy for some people:

Oh, the post-coital test, that is the worst one. Because of the distance of our clinic and the number of hours we were asked to leave between intercourse and test, we had to wake up at 3 a.m. Now have you ever tried getting excited when the alarm goes off at 3 a.m.? If it doesn't work, you've got to ring up the clinic and say, 'You know that appointment I had, well nothing happened.'

And what is the actual test like once everything has happened on schedule? 'It's just like having a cervical smear test once you get there. They are then able to see if the sperm are still alive. If they're not, they presume you have hostile mucus, then they have to inject the sperm into the womb past the cervical mucus.'

One more cynical patient comments, 'I sometimes think if they can't figure out anything else, they just say it's hostile mucus.' And the times it doesn't work?:

I was trying to see if my boyfriend and I had a problem, but I didn't really want to discuss it with him at that point. We had a fairly turbulent relationship and didn't live together and my biological time clock was ticking away. The lab was an hour away from home and only open during the day. My boyfriend worked in the Forestry Department, started work very early, and by the time he was home, it was too late to get to the clinic. I used to drive around with the lab order in my car and hope to find him for a private forest romp during the day and dash off to the lab. So to distract him from his work, I would have to wear the outfit he loved most on that particular day each month. It never worked. The one day he did come home early enough I bowled triumphantly into his house hoping for a warm reception only to find he had brought all his friends home for a beer. The table was surrounded by macho types. I beat a hasty retreat. I never did have the test done, we broke up soon afterwards.

―○―

The sperm test was easy to do, but not the post-coital. On one occasion, my husband went out for a drink after work. He phoned to say he would be back at about 9 p.m., but I said to enjoy himself and come back at 10 p.m. He got carried away and got home at midnight. I was furious, I threw a bottle of wine over him. I had worked myself up into a real state and felt he didn't care. I went to the doctor the next day having not had sex the night before so we were unable to do the test on that occasion. My husband rarely goes out on his own, this is not typical behaviour, but he would be naughty on the night it counted most.

Hystersalpingogram

The hystersalpingogram (HSG) is commonly called the dye test. This is one of the early tests for women to check the health and condition of the Fallopian tubes. My doctor advised me to take a couple of strong painkillers a couple of hours before, the type prescribed for period pain, and told me that I'd be fine to go to work after the test. So I didn't have any fears about it. However, the night before, a friend from New York came to stay. She, too, had been having fertility problems. I casually mentioned over dinner that I had to get up early the next day to go to the hospital for a test. Naturally she asked me what kind of test, as she'd already been through most of them. When I told her, she reacted with horror and told me her experience after the test.

She had the test on a Friday before a holiday weekend in New York and the test revealed blocked tubes. She hibernated for the weekend as her partner was away working, but started to feel very ill on the Sunday. An Australian friend was staying in the apartment below and came up to visit to be greeted by a very ill, rather green-looking friend. Being the sort of Australian who wouldn't give up, she rang all around New York to find a gynaecologist who would see our friend immediately. She was admitted to hospital very seriously ill with a tubal infection—the dye had not dispersed from her blocked tubes and she was in bad shape.

Now, I was absolutely riveted by this story, so naturally I then couldn't sleep. By the time I got to the X-ray department, I was rigid with fear. My doctor asked what the matter was—and was furious when I told him. 'Some friend,' he said.

My relatively painless test (a bit like a smear test with a sharp sting as the tube containing the dye went through the cervix) then filled me with wonder—I lay there dreading seeing some kind of blockage only to see these wonderful cobweb-like formations up on the screen, perfectly clear with dye streaming out the ends. I had no idea these tubes were so tiny and fragile. In all the diagrams I'd seen, they looked substantial, but as pointed out in the conception chapter, the diagrams are usually drawn from the outside, showing the exterior walls, not the interior, thread-size space. I felt huge relief and floated back to work. It was the first time I had been filled with awe for the minute mechanisms which carry new life. And it was only the beginning.

Many patients now have the laparoscopy and dye test — fondly referred to as a 'lap and dye' — done at the same time under a general anaesthetic.

Another, less positive view: 'I hated that test — I still think it is the worst experience of my life, the worst pain of my life.'

The Laparoscopy

This is the real day of reckoning for the woman, the day the doctor actually takes a small telescope and inserts it via a tiny cut near your navel into your gas-filled abdomen while you are under anaesthetic. From this imaging, the doctor can get a clear idea of the state of your reproductive system. He or she can see whether the ovaries and tubes are free of adhesions, the tiny cobweb-like strands that can form, particularly after previous surgery. He or she can see endometriosis, the condition where the womb lining sheds itself via the tubes into the stomach cavity and attaches itself to other organs, sometimes impeding normal function. The doctor can also see the shape and state of the uterus, and see if you have any fibroids, the pea-like tumours that can form in the muscles of the uterine wall. These are very common and, unless they are large, often cause no trouble at all.

I knew I'd had fibroids, as I'd had some removed during previous surgery. But I was quite upset when I was told by the doctor that I still had masses of small fibroids in my uterus. I went back to work the next day, but my stomach felt a bit battered and tender, and I had no idea it could contain so much wind.

Other women have had varied experiences and reactions to their laparoscopies. Some went back to work immediately, as I did; others took a weekend break. Some needed a week to recover:

'The laparoscopy hurt from referred pain in my shoulder for quite a few days. I also felt emotionally sore and abused by my circumstances. This was not fair. I was quite angry that I had to take time from work and explain why I had to go to hospital.

I also felt a lot of despair as this marked the time where I really had to admit to myself that I just wasn't going to fall pregnant on my own without a major miracle. I knew we were well on the road to seeking an assisted pregnancy. However, at this stage it still hadn't sunk in that we might not ever have a baby.'

'I felt quite good afterwards, compared to how I was told I might feel,' an English woman commented. 'I was taken great care of (Oh, for private treatment and not the NHS in England) and recovered quickly. But blocked tubes were the diagnosis.'

'I went in for a laparoscopy years ago and they said come back in six weeks and you'll be pregnant, not a problem. Can I have that in writing, nine years later?'

—∘—

'I felt bloated, sick and with a pain in my shoulders. It's OK when you're lying down still drowsy from the anaesthetic, but when you sit up all the gas rises and I felt like I was having a heart attack.'

Many reported they had been told they could go back to work the next day and simply didn't feel up to it. This problem is compounded when patients are having their tests secretly, so explanations of time off work and hospital visits become another problem, like the following woman:

I was told I'd just need just one day off work and we booked a Friday off work so I could have the weekend to follow. I was told it didn't involve anything other than two small nicks and a general anaesthetic. When I came out of the anaesthetic I was in agony. I could see there was blood on one side of the gown and I couldn't see where it was coming from; I later worked out it was from the laparoscopy. I had two stitches in my tummy, just below the navel, and couldn't even stand up straight. They mentioned in passing the pain you can expect in your shoulder blades because of the gas used and handed me some painkillers and an appointment card. I was very unprepared for that experience. I had a week off work and had to explain I'd been in hospital for tests, which then involved telling them what the problem was.

Some people feel that the operation's outcome determines how well they feel:

I'd been on a DI [donor insemination] program for six months and nothing had happened so they decided I should have a laparoscopy. I did feel lousy—but more because they didn't find anything. I was really hoping they'd find something and fix it up and we'd be able to get on with it. I didn't find the after-effects of the exploratory laparoscopy too bad, but had a later laparoscopy when we did a cycle of GIFT treatment and when they said none of the remaining eggs had fertilised, all of a sudden the after-effects became worse.

Fortunately for those living in Australia, there aren't the waiting lists or the lack of availability of tests on Medicare, the public health system. Also, most couples take out private health insurance to bridge the cost gaps. However, for those in other countries, where private health insurance isn't usual, the family budget has to be considered. One couple in the United Kingdom, who had wanted a baby for many years, had this experience:

We live in York in the UK and our local hospital doesn't have a fertility unit so we had to go quite a distance. In our area, the National Health Service wouldn't pay *for treatment, so we had to go to a private hospital and pay for everything, without any extra health insurance. The wonderful doctor there eventually managed to get us on her list at the NHS hospital with a good fertility clinic. Somehow, she managed to squeeze us in on her NHS list — initially she told us we'd have to pay and that would have been about £1200 [about $2400] for the day in hospital. We would have had to save for that or take a loan out. Because I'm a bit overweight, she warned me that they mightn't be able to get into my tummy, but in the end there was no problem with that. It showed my tubes were both clear, although there is a little wobble in one of them, but not enough to stop a sperm getting through. So another worry was gone.*

Blood Tests

Through the use of blood tests, the fertility clinic tracks the various hormone levels throughout the cycle and make sure the luteinizing hormone produces its required surge to push out the egg and that the oestrogen and progesterone levels are normal for the stage of the cycle. These tests are often referred to as hormone assays, and also review prolactin levels to see if this breastfeeding hormone is present in too high a quantity.

An AIDS (HIV) test is now universal for everyone before they can undergo fertility treatment. Also, doctors will check for rubella immunity to make sure a woman's schoolgirl vaccination is still valid, as rubella, or German measles, can still be a disaster in the first months of pregnancy. Tests are also done for hepatitis B.

Test Results

The ways we are told our test results vary with the personalities of our medical consultants. To tell a couple they have a major problem isn't easy for anyone. Professor Robert Jansen, director of Sydney IVF, says the only way to do it is to be 'frank, gentle, don't ascribe blame. And most importantly, to allow a lot of time with the couple during that appointment.'

My first fertility specialist was very blunt and brusque in his approach, but Dr Steigrad was direct and down-to-earth, telling us the sperm weren't great and I had multiple fibroids, but he told us in a non-dramatic, calm way, and then told us what we should do next. I think the important thing all couples suggest they need after a negative diagnosis of any kind is the pathway laid out for them to follow. That somehow takes the immediate emotional sting away, and gives you something positive upon which to focus.

Others tell of their responses to tests results:

Because I worked in a lab, when I looked at my husband's sperm count I said, 'Oh, I see the problem.' I was upset, but as we weren't hopeless to conceive naturally, we still felt positive we could achieve a natural pregnancy. Then when that seemed unlikely, I thought OK, I've got a problem, how am I going to fix it?

I applied for adoption, I read up everything on assisted fertility, got the name of a specialist and thought, right, let's attack this.

~·~

After two years of testing me, they finally tested my husband to find he was producing no sperm at all. I hadn't had good experiences at that hospital, so it was in keeping that they told us fairly coldly that my problems were not important, it was the fact there were no sperm that mattered. They said we had three choices: to give up there and then, to apply for adoption, or to have further tests on my husband.

I remember crying all the way back to work, picking jobs all afternoon that meant I wasn't on my own. On the way home I stopped and bought Marc a single red rose and a card to tell him we would face it together. I was absolutely devastated, and looking back, he went into shock. He was doing his final exams at university and this was the last thing he needed.

Because we live in England, we had to wait a further twelve months for another test: they said he had primary testicular failure and there was no treatment at all. At this point, donor insemination was discussed, but there was a two-year wait for treatment. They said they would have liked to offer us further counselling, but no funds were available! It was at this point I didn't know how we were going to cope. Marc was having trouble accepting the diagnosis and didn't feel the fertility issue affected him at all. We eventually found a DI clinic that was convenient and affordable. We finally achieved a pregnancy only to have our hopes dashed at thirteen weeks when the baby miscarried. The hospital, a different one, was superb. We were referred to the foetal centre to find out why we lost our baby, and it was through not telling them that the baby was conceived from DI that my husband was given a genetic test. He was shown to have an extra chromosome — Klinefelter's syndrome — which means no sperm are present in these people. This diagnosis has changed his life. He is a completely different person, he has an answer. This has given him the courage to tell his family and friends.

~·~

My husband had a vasectomy reversal done as soon as we wanted to start a family. The specialist told us the sperm count wasn't good and sent us back to the urologist for another reversal. The urologist sent us back saying the reversal was fine, the sperm weren't though. Someone told us that if the vasectomy reversal is done within a couple of years of the original operation, it is usually successful. But he said that as my husband's vasectomy was eleven or twelve years ago, it could cause a problem. Apparently the body can build up a hostility to its own sperm. The immune system tries to fight them off as though they were foreign bodies. They come out in stuff like Super Glue, they can't go anywhere. We have a friend who had some medical knowledge, so he actually stored some of his sperm before he had his vasectomy, he even bought his own sperm bank container and brought it over here from England. He now has a baby through GIFT treatment from his stored sperm.

~·~

My husband also had a vasectomy reversal, but no one told us to start trying immediately for a baby as the scar tissue could block the tube again.

⁓

All the investigations found nothing was wrong with us. Every time we go to the clinic they say there is nothing wrong with us. Nine years later ... You've got nothing solid to talk with people about when they tell you their diagnosis, nothing to work on.

⁓

They found I had endometriosis all around one ovary, so with that and my husband's poor sperm count, we have a lot of problems.

Through this testing, the fertility specialist gets a clear picture of your case, except for those with unexplained infertility. The blood test for progesterone levels will confirm that you are ovulating. The temperature chart will indicate the duration of the cycle and its luteal phase, the time after ovulation has taken place. This second half of the cycle, which is more consistent than the first (pre-ovulatory phase), varies from ten to seventeen days in 95 per cent of women.

The 'quality' of the ovulation is assessed by the duration of the luteal phase, the quality of the endometrium (lining of the womb) and the measurement of the progesterone levels (which indicate whether the corpus luteum is functioning normally to build up the uterine lining for the implantation of a pregnancy). So, even if the temperature taking is boring, it does form a useful purpose in the early stages of fertility investigation.

The semen analysis is usually called a sperm count, but this is an incomplete description of this test. Not only will the laboratory want to test for the numbers of sperm present, but they will also test for their motility (ability to swim) and their appearance (whether they are normal or abnormal, alive or dead).

The post-coital test will tell the clinic whether the sperm can perform effectively in the woman's mucus, or whether there is a mucus hostility present.

The hystersalpingogram or dye test, as explained, will show whether a woman's tubes are clear for the free flow of sperm and egg — and conception if it takes place.

The laparoscopy will give doctors a clear picture of a woman's reproductive organs. They will make sure the uterus is normal, the ovaries are free of endometriosis or adhesions, and the tubes are free to move across and collect the eggs when they are ovulated.

Of all the conditions revealed by these tests, ovulation problems can be the simplest to solve, simply requiring drug therapy to stimulate the ovaries into response. Most of the other problems revealed in these tests, however, will need help from assisted reproductive technology.

Chapter 6
Out-of-Body Pregnancy Procedures

Assisted Reproductive Technology and
In Vitro Fertilisation

'My best moment of infertility came in the early days of despair.
My husband is one of six children and I am the eldest of five. My parents
are divorced and at that time things were still bitter between them and my mother
was quick to lay anything awful at my father's doorstep. She was asking about our
problems and trying to make sense of the madness when we both obviously came
from such fertile backgrounds. Finally she threw her hands in the air and said:
"Well it must come from your father's side because I have five children."
However, her smug look faded as I reminded her that he
had fathered those same five children.'

~

'Some people are fascinated by IVF when you tell them, but nobody really
has any idea what is involved with an IVF cycle. Every day they ask, "What did you
do today ... when's your next cycle ..."'

~

'Our support group was raising money and someone actually
asked, "What are infertile people?" I said, "I'm one of them." Someone else
got us mixed up with the HIV group, they muddled the initials. I wish we
made as much money as that group does.'

The term *assisted reproductive technology* embraces a whole field of fertility assistance
pioneered by Dr Patrick Steptoe and Dr Robert Edwards in England and Professor Carl
Wood's team in Melbourne, Australia. Each year the techniques are further refined to
help couples who, up until 1978, would have remained childless. Even when GIFT was
discussed with me in the late 1980s, the risk of large multiple births was still great. Now
doctors put back just three eggs or embryos, so that risk has been practically eliminated.

The list of treatments features a fascinating group of acronyms, sometimes referred
to as 'IVF-speak', denoting often unpronounceable medical terms. The following is a
brief run-down of the most common ones, but you *must* ask your doctor to explain the
treatment that is suggested for you.

IVF (IN VITRO FERTILISATION) Literally fertilisation in glass, these conceptions occur when the sperm and eggs are combined in a test tube. If the egg and sperm combine successfully, and form viable embryos, a maximum of three embryos is placed directly into the uterus, by-passing the (presumably damaged) Fallopian tubes. There it is hoped at least one of the embryos will continue to develop and burrow into the uterine lining to create a pregnancy.

GIFT (GAMETE INTRA-FALLOPIAN TRANSFER) Eggs are collected from the woman by laparoscopy or trans-vaginally by ultrasound guidance, and placed directly into the Fallopian tube with the sperm, which has been collected and treated in the laboratory to give the best possible sample. The replacement procedure is done with a fine sterile tube. This treatment is more natural than in vitro fertilisation in that the egg and sperm are given the maximum chance to merge naturally, and travel down the tube and implant naturally in the uterus. Of course, the tubes must be clear for this to be advised. (*Gamete* is a generic word that refers to any germ cell. So it refers to the egg in the female; the sperm in the male.)

ZIFT (ZYGOTE INTRA-FALLOPIAN TRANSFER) This is a similar procedure to the above, except the egg and sperm are combined in the laboratory and the resulting conception, the zygote, is replaced into the tube for the natural journey down the Fallopian tube into the uterus for implantation.

ICSI (pronounced ik-sy) This is a relatively new procedure used when the sperm is deficient and cannot penetrate the egg on its own. A single sperm is injected into the centre of the egg. The advent of this technique was a major advancement for couples where the husband was producing some sperm, but these sperm were too feeble or immature to fertilise an egg unaided. Couples who would have otherwise been advised to seek donor insemination or adoption to create their families now have some hope of a genetic child created by both partners.

BOOST These letters originally stood for buserelin oocyte stimulation treatment, but the drug buserelin has now been largely replaced by other drugs. The drug, part of a group of drugs known as GnRH analogues, is used to create a surge of hormones from the pituitary gland, which generates the production of many follicles. Other drugs are also added for several days then an injection of hCG (human chorionic gonadotrophin, an essential hormone which encourages final maturing of follicles) is given, followed by egg pick-up in 36 hours. This is followed by fertilisation of eggs in the laboratory and replacement in the woman's uterus.

DOWN REGULATION This is a method of controlling the events in a cycle. A combination of drugs shuts down the natural messages from the pituitary gland to the ovary. Drugs are used as in BOOST treatment, but over a longer period.

NATURAL CYCLE   So called when any of the assisted reproductive technologies are used, but the procedures are done without drug therapy in a normal menstrual cycle.

FROZEN CYCLE   This is when stored frozen embryos from another treatment cycle are thawed and replaced into the uterus without the need for egg stimulation and pick-up.

SUZI (SUB-ZONAL INSEMINATION)   This involves placing the sperm under the outer shell of the egg using a microscope and special equipment, if the sperm are too weak to penetrate the shell. This has largely been replaced by ICSI.

MICRODROP INSEMINATION   The sperm is prepared so only a very small amount of fluid surrounds it. The egg and sperm are then combined as with usual IVF.

These are just a few of the most common terms now used under the collective term of IVF. If you think a new branch of the English language has been born, you are probably right. Most clinics will have some written information to introduce you to the world of assisted reproduction.

The first appointment with your specialist will probably generate a head full of questions once you leave the surgery or clinic. You may want to ask if you can tape-record your appointments, so you can refer later to things you don't understand. Or you may wish to take notes. The most important thing is that you understand what your treatment will be, why you are having it and how to implement whatever drugs you are given. What not to do:

> *We have so many funny things in our refrigerator ... injections, oestrogen pessaries. Because my name is in our newsletter as a support telephone number, a woman rang one night to ask me if she took her pessaries with water. 'No,' I said, 'you take them with mucus.' Then she asked, 'Do you stick one up each nostril?' She even asked if you took the alfoil off! I rang the clinic to see if they'd explained the treatment to her properly and they said they'd just got off the phone with her, and even then she rang me.*

The (More) Natural Way

Before the refinement and relative success of IVF treatment, women with blocked tubes had only one hope — that the doctor could clear or repair their damaged tubes. I asked Dr Steigrad if tubal surgery was still a valid treatment, as I'd read in some British research that many doctors there now prefer to go straight on to IVF. This was his answer.

> *Basically we still do reconstructive surgery. You need to look carefully at the problem and also at the age of the patient. And then you give them the options. It is interesting that people used to say that if the patient was older there really*

wasn't time for reconstructive surgery. But equally the pregnancy rates from IVF with older patients is pretty appalling.

Interestingly, recently at an international fertility conference in France there were two presentations where doctors had taken patients who had been on IVF unsuccessfully, had performed reconstructive surgery on them, and these patients had conceived naturally, and they were in their early 40s. So there is the suggestion that IVF may not be the greatest thing for this group, it certainly doesn't have a high pregnancy rate....

We also have an in-between stage where we do a controlled ovarian stimulation program for patients who have no known cause of infertility. With these patients we are giving them three cycles of controlled hyper-stimulation [of eggs] with natural intercourse and are getting very high pregnancy rates indeed. And for patients with no problems in the women and mild male factor [poor sperm], we are combining the controlled hyper-stimulation program with intra-uterine insemination of washed sperm and achieving good results.

This is a halfway house between saying there is nothing we can do for you and the only thing we can do for you is IVF. This is probably a group of patients who would become pregnant very quickly on IVF, so it lowers the percentage statistics on IVF and GIFT treatments, but it is good as it doesn't involve the operative egg pick-up. But patients experience the controlled stimulation as with IVF and it sometimes makes it easier if the decision is made for them to slide on to IVF treatment or not. If they over-respond to controlled stimulation cycle, we can convert that to an IVF cycle anyway, so we have a built-in safety factor.

Starting treatment

Between your appointment with the specialist to discuss the treatment you will receive and your first treatment cycle, many clinics have an information night where couples gather to have treatments explained and ask questions. The following reactions are typical:

I think we all felt so excited after that initial information night that we thought it was going to happen with the first cycle, so we didn't need to know any more.

Our basic queries were answered during an information night before we began treatment. These are great, however, I think it would benefit a couple more if they were to attend a second one as you are apt to go away from the first one in a state of euphoria and excitement, and fresh questions surface after a couple of days.

Dr Steigrad concluded:

There is no doubt in my mind that if I have an educated [in fertility] patient who understands what we are trying to do they can actually assist because they understand, and certainly their level of stress goes down substantially if we say this is what we are going to do and this is why we are doing it. I've discovered patients who have had two or three cycles of IVF elsewhere and in my preliminary interview with them it becomes obvious they have huge gaps, even though they have actually experienced the cycles. We've then put the brakes on and gone back to square one and arranged for them to go through a full counselling process and I think there hasn't been one who hasn't appreciated the time — losing in fact a bit of time — but taking the time to understand what it's all about, how this happens and the mechanisms. It makes a huge difference.

Logistics

From now until the time you are successfully pregnant, you will probably feel you are attached to your clinic by a kind of umbilical cord. However, to get through treatment successfully, you must work out *how* you are going to manage your life and incorporate your fertility clinic.

You will need to attend for blood tests to check the levels of your hormones, injections of hormones (if you don't feel your husband or nearby relative or friend can be trained to do this), ultrasound scans to assess the progress of your egg-forming follicles and you have to anticipate dropping everything at the time you are told your eggs will be ready for collection, fertilisation and replacement.

If you are going to succeed, these things have to be worked out in advance, to reduce the stress when you are actually going through a cycle.

Depending on your particular work and your relationship with your employer, you have to make a decision whether to confide in them or not. Because I'd had two miscarriages and had to have some time off work, our then-publisher Richard Walsh did know I wanted a baby and that I was having treatment at a fertility clinic. As a trained doctor, he was very supportive and concerned that I take time off from work next time I succeeded in conceiving. But as a publisher he was anxiously trying to make me find a replacement for myself if and when that time came.

I found this extremely stressful. I was confused and felt a failure in my inability to hold on to a pregnancy. I was in no way sure I would ever be successful. I loved my job and certainly didn't want to surrender it on the mere chance that this mythical baby might come. Yet I also understood (sort of) his wish and need to be organised in a commercial sense. But once people knew I was trying to have a baby, I felt each month of failure more keenly as it was under the spotlight. I am much better at dealing with anguish privately. Only you, the patient, can decide what is best in your circumstances.

Some husbands are pleased to be involved and, while they don't actually relish the idea of giving injections to the woman they love, except a sadistic few ('I've always enjoyed playing darts'), they can learn and this saves her rushing off to the clinic at odd times.

'We were fortunate enough to have an Accident and Emergency Centre at our local hospital open all hours for blood tests and injections,' said a Gold Coast woman. 'I often found myself there after I finished work at 10.30 p.m. This fitted easily into the program and wasn't stressful at all.'

CAROLYN, A NURSE, TELLS HOW HER HUSBAND WAS TRAINED TO GIVE HER THE INJECTIONS SHE NEEDED:

Just before we were about to embark on our first cycle, we had an appointment with the nurse who works with our professor. It was she who taught Bruce and I went along as well. He has never done anything like that before and was happy to help, but wasn't greatly looking forward to it. The nurse actually has a plastic model of someone's torso, say from ribs down to the top of thighs. It shows tummy, belly button down to pubic area and it also has a bottom on it. Presumably that little model has taken thousands of injections over the past few years.

First she explained to both of us how to draw up the injection. There are two forms of injection, one is subcutaneous, meaning it goes just under the skin and the place it goes is in the nice little soft pad just about all of us have in the middle of our tummies, around, but not too close to the belly button. So what you do is squeeze it with two fingers and you just pop the injection in. It's a very tiny needle and very short, and you don't put a lot of fluid into it. So she showed him how to do those, and with a lot of the injections we had to mix two drugs, and some of them come in powder form, and you have to know how to mix those. You get sterile water with it, then you mix that with the other drug. So she showed us all that and then she gave him a couple of practices with the subcutaneous ones. That's the best one to start on really because you can't do too much harm. Especially in that area where it is just going into fat *[laugh]*. The majority of the injections are these — say if you are prescribed twelve injections in a cycle, you might have eight that are this type.

The last few are intra-muscular or IM, and the best spot is your bottom. You divide one cheek (buttock) into four and you take the upper outer quadrant and that's where you put it. With that one, the nurse told him that's where to put it, but with my nursing knowledge, I know that's how you miss the sciatic nerve. She didn't tell Bruce that, which is probably good, but being the person who was going to receive the injection, I was quite keen he was going to miss my sciatic nerve so I pointed that out to him. These ones he didn't enjoy — he didn't enjoy it at all — but those ones he didn't relish, where the other ones weren't quite so — well traumatic is too strong a word — anxiety-inducing perhaps.

With the first ones it would be just sitting in a lounge chair, popped in and gone. With the other ones, it would be lying down on the bed face down and then I can't even see that he's in the right area. That was a little bit more 'yucky'. So he was taught by the nurse. Was he nervous? Yes, just wanting to be sure he was doing the right thing. Also the fact that he was giving it to me, whom he loves, and knowing that I knew exactly where it should go, and from my point of view, he hadn't even had the training a student nurse would have. But he was taught the right spot and he got it every time. The injections in your bottom do hurt, so for me it wasn't great, but I tried not to make a fuss about it, because it wasn't nice for him either, having to inflict it on me. Again, remembering this is something you are in together, you are doing it for something you both want to achieve, it's not one person inflicting it on the other. You are doing it because you love each other if that doesn't sound funny.

When travelling, there are a few precautions to follow:

We were taking a little break and going off to Bali for a week and I was a bit concerned about going through Customs with all these little bottles and things. I asked the clinic and they said you should advise the end of the flight sector that you have these things, and leave armed with a prescription and proof of treatment from the clinic, otherwise, don't go, especially to Asian countries.

~

With the IVF injections I felt unable to inject myself, as did my husband, so we had to get a variety of doctors from my local practice to do it daily. This was fine while I was at home, but on one occasion I was called away during a long weekend and the clinic had given me no treatment card or written proof of the program. The only doctor available refused to do it, and only agreed once he telephoned my own doctor, at home, on the holiday Monday. So the moral of that story is, make sure you have some medical instructions in case you are called away from home during a cycle.

~

Starting a cycle

The doctors all talk about having realistic expectations of treatment and not putting your life on hold, but few patients manage to remain cool and calm at this time of major upheaval, physical and mental. As one woman put it:

I remember talking to another woman in the waiting room before my first attempt. I was so excited I was practically blowing up balloons and she was on her thirteenth attempt, and very cynical. She said things like, 'You'll be back, you'll see.' I remember saying, 'No, I won't.' She was right.

Her friend commented: 'Even the nurses are like that, they say you can keep this drug for your next attempt, and you think there's not going to be another one.'

Dr Steigrad comments on those expectations:

It all comes down to having realistic expectations. That makes non-success less traumatic. The trouble is people will talk about success and failure. And they look at not getting pregnant that cycle as failure. And it's not failure, it's nature. You say there is a 20 per cent pregnancy rate which means there will be an 80 per cent non-pregnancy rate. All patients believe they will be in that first 20 per cent. You've got to believe it.

As I didn't have IVF, I have to rely on fellow patients sharing their experiences of an IVF cycle. There will be as many experiences as there are patients, but Carolyn, the nurse who explained her injections, takes us through her first cycle.

Bruce is my husband's name. We've been married since 1988. In 1989, we discovered that my husband had testicular cancer — he had an operation and had one testicle removed and had five lots of chemotherapy after this. We were told basically that after the chemo, it would be at least three years before his sperm would be viable to form a child. He tried to put sperm into storage, but the sperm turned out to be no good. So we knew we had a bit of a wait ahead of us. As it turned out, I was ready long before Bruce to start a family, but he wasn't probably until the end of 1994. I stopped taking the Pill at that stage, and at the beginning of 1995 we started officially trying for a child. He'd been having regular check-ups with his oncologist all along, and they were all good reports, but we realised things may not happen very quickly.

By August 1995, at his regular check-up with his oncologist, I asked him to have a sperm sample done. He was a little more reluctant, but the oncologist said tests are a dime a dozen, go for it. So it showed that he had some good sperm, but his count was certainly low and not all of them were good.

After the results of that, the oncologist referred us to one of the professors at Monash IVF, and I think we saw him first in November for a few tests, then in January for a sperm count, and a few more blood tests for both of us. In January, he also told us he wanted me to have a laparoscopy as that was a routine part of his treatment. We asked if it was really worth going through all of this, but we decided it was better to know now, rather than to drag on with it.

I had my laparoscopy, D&C and dye test late in January and was quite shocked to learn I had very bad adhesions around my tubes and the doctor gave me a 20 per cent chance of conceiving if there hadn't been any problems with Bruce. As you can imagine, with his low sperm count, his chances were certainly lower than 20 per cent, but we both thought we'll give it a go.

We didn't have to wait any time to get on the waiting list by the time we were ready to start IVF. My period came on the first of May and we got into it. I told friends that I was certainly excited and interested to see how it was going to go. I remember saying I will be a lot wiser in a month's time. Well it was actually two months that signalled my first getting of wisdom. I learned a lot in these two months.

First of all, there are a few different ways to have IVF — the one I was on was called BOOST, so on day 1 you had to have the full flow of your period by 6 p.m. and ring the clinic and say you are calling this day 1.

They give you a little table to tell you when to start your drugs. The two drugs I had to have subcutaneously, mixed together in the same syringe were Lucrin and Metrodin. You have to have Lucrin for a day before Metrodin begins. They also work it out so they don't have to do any egg pick-ups on a Sunday, which is practical from an operative point of view. My day 1 was a Wednesday, so I didn't have anything.

Day 2, 2 May, again I had nothing.

Day 3 I had a Lucrin injection subcutaneously.

Day 4 I had Lucrin and Metrodin mixed together. This continued till day 9 when I had a blood test to determine how my hormones were responding and that would then determine if I needed a bigger dose of either or both of the drugs. At this time, I also had a vaginal ultrasound to see if enough follicles were growing to warrant an egg pick-up in a few days time. In my case, both those things were fine, so I continued the same dosage of the two drugs.

On Day 11, I had another blood test and the levels were going up nicely, so I had to continue with the same dosage.

Day 12 marked the last day of the subcutaneous injections.

On Day 13, I had to have my first intramuscular injection, that had to be exactly 36 hours before egg pick-up was due. So this was scheduled for 9.30 a.m. on the 15 May, so I had to have my Profasi intra-muscular injection 36 hours earlier at 9.30 p.m. on Day 13.

Then you don't have the subcutaneous injections any more.

I went into hospital at 8.15 a.m. on 15 May. My husband had to be there for an 8.30 appointment to give his sperm specimen.

I had to fast for the egg pick-up. It's not a full anaesthetic, but they put you out because it is not totally pleasant. Getting the sperm sample isn't the easiest thing in life, I do feel for Bruce. The times we've gone in to give the actual sperm sample to make the baby we've actually caught the train, so tangling with public transport before we get there, we are not exactly relaxed. In our clinic, you sort of have to perform in this small room — it's not your own home and it's not comfortable and the couch fits about a five-year-old child, not two grown adults — it doesn't exactly help you to relax, but we got both the sperm samples out.

We did find it hard to do it in an unnatural way and setting.

They say you need to ejaculate three times in the previous eight days, then you have to have three days of abstinence before you give your sperm donation.

The first sample there didn't seem to be very much, so we wondered if some had gone inside me. I went off to have my egg pick-up, which meant I'd been sedated. Then after that we had to do another sperm specimen as the first one wasn't good enough. I was just a little bit groggy, not terrible, but I certainly wasn't feeling like having to do that a second time, and neither was my husband.

With the ejaculate, they can do micro-drop and micro-injection. Ours was micro-drop, so there is not a lot of fluid around the sperm and egg as they are trying to get together. It doesn't have to travel too far.

Egg pick-up was at 9.30 a.m. on 15 May and the day after you ring up to see if any of your eggs have fertilised and to work out when you are going to have them put back.

I had seven eggs picked up and five fertilised, so I had enough to put back.

On 17 May, I went in at 9.45 a.m. and had my embryos put back at 10.45 a.m. They actually show you a photo taken through a microscope of the three embryos, or however many you choose, so you can see. They say this is a four-cell one, this is an eight-cell one, this is a six-cell one. Then you need some booster injections of the same drug intramuscularly. So on day 19 and day 23 I had those

A couple of days after you have the embryos put back, you can ring the clinic and see if there are any embryos left (which continued developing), and you can have them frozen. But ours were not suitable for freezing.

After that is the killer waiting period to see if they have implanted. I found out on 31 May that I was pregnant. Then you have to wait two weeks and when you are medically six weeks pregnant you have a vaginal ultrasound and that is where the rot set in my first cycle, and the joy came in my second.

We had prepared ourselves that it could go either way and things didn't normally happen the first time, so we were both pretty staggered when I was pregnant. We had told (as well as both sets of parents) five couples who are obviously our closest friends.

On the day I found out I was pregnant, the professor did ring me and say my blood hormone levels were low, and to be cautiously optimistic and have a blood test in another week. By the time I had that blood test, it was still a bit low. He repeated to be cautiously optimistic and have a blood test and ultrasound at what would be six weeks pregnant.

The six-week ultrasound showed that either there was nothing there or it was a week behind — basically it was pretty blank. The doctor who did that ultrasound was extremely kind; I was pouring tears right, left and centre. He said there was probably no more than a 30 per cent chance that the baby was still there. I had noticed in the time that I was pregnant my breasts were quite tender and I had an absolute absence of pimples — normally I have one or two a week, however, about three days before my ultrasound I noticed that my breasts had gone down. On the day of the ultrasound, I was absolutely devastated for about three hours when I got home, and we had to ring our friends and give them the bad news — or say that it wasn't looking too good. We had to wait about ten days after that ultrasound to have a second ultrasound to see if it was delayed growth or if there was nothing there. I remember asking Bruce could he sedate me for the next ten days because I just couldn't see how I'd get through it. I did — as you know, time just goes on regardless. By the second ultrasound I should have been 7$^{1}/_{2}$ weeks pregnant. The sac was still growing, but there was nothing in it — so my body was telling itself I was pregnant, but I wasn't. That was a Monday, I saw the professor that afternoon and on the following Thursday I had a D&C. So out of the two-month period, the first month, the official treatment cycle, was the easy bit; the second, the waiting and the emotional trauma were absolute killers.

I think everyone would agree the waiting and your brain going over and over are the things that really kill you, not the treatment. I haven't actually found the treatment that difficult, though I can't say I enjoy the injections.

Two or three weeks after the D&C were not fantastic. I would say we both coped very well, I am still emotional about it. It was classed as a silent miscarriage — it could have taken two days or it could have taken three weeks before my body expelled the sac. I sort of lost it for a few days and then for the next weeks I probably cried a few times a week when someone would say something that would just set me off, regardless of whether it was about IVF or not.

We regard ourselves as very lucky because our second IVF attempt also resulted in a pregnancy, and this pregnancy seems to be progressing normally, though we were very cautious at first.

Another patient, Jacqueline, kept a diary of her first treatment cycle using ICSI. Here is her story:

We always knew there would be a problem as my husband Greg had already been married and had two children and a vasectomy. But not long after we were married, he went to see a urologist and he had an operation to have his vasectomy reversed. They did a sperm count after the operation and said everything was fine.

Greg lost his job not long after this, so we decided to wait until he was employed again before we tried to have a baby. We tried for a year and nothing happened, so we went to see our doctor. Another sperm count revealed there was nothing coming through, the vasectomy had closed up again. We were so angry no one had told us this was a likely option and that we should have tried immediately after the vasectomy reversal was done.

The fertility specialist we were advised to see did a routine laparoscopy on me and found I had severe endometriosis, especially around the ovaries. He advised us that IVF was our only chance. We both had trouble coming to terms with that. We still hoped by some miracle that we may conceive naturally. I asked the doctor what he would advise me to do if I was his daughter. He explained to me how the ovaries and tubes have to be unrestricted to function properly. And we still had Greg's problem.

Our professor invited us to an information night and also gave us a long appointment where he explained our options. He told us about the ICSI program, and how they could inject sperm that were not very good into the egg and conceive successfully. He gave me a stack of things to read about the program, and said we could start the next week if we wanted to. But Greg took some time in coming round to the idea that nothing was going to happen naturally. A few months later he was ready, and our professor arranged an appointment with another fertility specialist for us as he wanted to give us another opinion. This doctor was great, too, though she did seem in a bit of a rush. But because Greg was still unsure at this point, I felt it was very important for her to help answer his questions.

I began treatment with one month of sniffing Syranel — they say this is good for the endometriosis. Luckily we went to Bali for the first two weeks. I had bad headaches every day. I still do now, but you get used to them. I felt the clinic had forgotten me and it would have been nice to have a phone call or even a note in the mail to see how I was going.

12 November   After one month of taking my Synarel nasal spray, I am finally ready to have the blood test to see if we are ready to take the next step. The nurse was great and told me what I will be doing and what to expect. My phone call later in the day gave me the good answer I was praying for.

13 November   Today is the first day of my injections. I am more nervous than I have ever been (about the same as on my wedding day). By the time I got to the clinic and waited — thank God it was only 10 minutes and not 45 like yesterday — I was a nervous wreck. The sister was great and tried to calm me down and talked me through the whole thing. After she had finished, I had to agree it was not so bad. When I returned to my car all I wanted to do was cry. So many things, emotions. I wished Greg was here and not overseas with his work. Will we one day be lucky enough to have our own baby? It just seems such a long path from trying to fall pregnant to this point (18 months).

19 November   Almost one week of injections at the clinic and I don't care what anyone says, they do hurt and your arm hurts for the rest of the day. I had my blood test and the results showed I still had a way to go. I am very happy with the nursing staff, they make you feel good about it all.

22 November   By now I am feeling really fat, tired, irritable and always thirsty. Today's blood test showed that my levels had dropped rather than increased. The decision was made to increase my doses. On the ultrasound I could see what was happening.

26 November   I am so tired now, but other patients say this is normal. My blood test results were good and they decided that tomorrow I have my last injection plus my big needle tomorrow night ready for theatre. On today's ultrasound, the nurse was showing me the follicles that the eggs live in (no wonder I feel fat).

28 November   By lunch time today, I decided I really shouldn't have come to work (but I stayed anyway). I am feeling very tired and had a very sore stomach. At least they will come out tomorrow.

29 November   This morning I was feeling really bad. I was wheeled to theatre at 8 a.m. My doctor came and spoke to me and explained he was very concerned with the way my levels had been changing. He was concerned they might not find anything. As the anaesthetist was preparing, the doctor spoke nice words to me and at this moment I thought I am very happy with him and do trust him. When I awoke the first thing I did was look at my hand. It said 6 (6 eggs) and I was upset as I didn't think this was enough, but I was reassured by the nurses in recovery that this was the average. Greg gave his semen donation and then it was home to take it easy and wait for the call in the morning to see if they fertilised.

30 November   Two hours after they said the scientist would phone we still hadn't heard. I made the phone call then. The scientist was very nice and explained that the sperm wasn't any good and that none of the eggs had fertilised. Since that moment I have had an ache in my heart. It feels like someone very close to me has died. I have done so much thinking and I keep asking the question what do we do now? We are booked in to see the professor in two weeks. We will be totally guided by what he says. I feel like he has my life in his hands and in a way he does, because if we can't do anything else, I do not want to live my life without a child.

Two months later she adds: It is amazing that life goes on. I am now two weeks into my second cycle and am sniffing the Synarel twice a day. Really your life revolves around the treatment. We saw the doctor and he told me he had difficulty retrieving my eggs as the endometriosis had become worse and was surrounding the eggs. This time when they operate on me to remove my eggs, they will also operate on Greg and remove some hopefully good sperm where they are made.

  I don't really talk to anyone about the hurt that I have experienced and am feeling. Little things upset me. My sister is now pregnant and mum and dad are ecstatic. I am so happy for her, but it hurts so much, not that I say anything to her or the family. The pain I felt on the Saturday when I heard that my eggs hadn't fertilised and, worse still, that Greg's sperm was no good was the worst I have felt so far in my life. I don't believe Greg will ever experience the hurt and sometimes anger I feel as he already has his two children.

Chapter 7
Coping with Treatment

Success in fertility treatment often equals staying power.

Not many patients are *first time lucky*. So staying intact physically, emotionally and socially are critical if you have to withstand many treatment cycles. There is no magic potion which you can drink to remain eternally positive and optimistic. A sense of humour helps. Good support from your medical team helps. Helping each other helps. And joining a support group where you can share the good, the bad and the funny experiences can give great strength in what is otherwise a very lonely quest. It will change your life forever. And your relationship with your partner and others.

Psychologists say people dig into their deepest interior when confronted with birth, death and divorce (and maybe moving house). With infertility treatment, each month brings a microcosm of all those things — to be experienced, dealt with, put aside, then begun all over again in the next treatment cycle.

Putting Your Life on Hold

Every doctor and member of the clinic staff will tell you not to put your life *on hold*, to do everything as normally as possible and try to fit in your infertility treatment around other areas of your home and work. In theory, few patients would disagree. Most patients would agree, however, that it is impossible. You are focused in such an intense way on your body, and you are aware the actions of this cycle, if successful, can change your life forever. So you can't really pretend it isn't happening. Here are ways some patients have dealt with this:

> *'Because I live in far northern Queensland [Australia], we either had to go to the clinic in Brisbane, or a satellite clinic in Townsville. That is still a 400-kilometre round trip, so you really had to take your holidays and stay down there for the critical period. I was involved in IVF for three years, so all our holidays for three years were centred on IVF, so that's hardly living a normal life.'*

> *'You do put your life on hold, there is nothing you can do without wondering do I do X or keep on trying to have a baby? Do we spend the money on a renovation, or do we spend it on IVF? You keep trying to stay positive,'* said a woman from Sydney, Australia.

> *'It does affect your whole life,'* responded another. *'You work out that you may have failed this month, but you'll try again in six months time, so that's all you're thinking about, six months down the track. In the meantime, you just keep on going to work, waiting, because we did have to wait six months between clinics in Northern Queensland. I found the waiting seemed longer each time.'*

> *'The hardest thing is that in our clinic in Sydney they tell you to get on with the rest of your life normally, but how can they know what it is like? Not one of the doctors or staff have been through infertility treatment themselves, they can't possibly understand. To you it's the biggest thing in the world, this treatment, and it has cost you a fortune. Sometimes they seem very matter-of-fact about it all.'*

Even the most trivial thing is hard to organise — like your wardrobe if you are the editor of a fashion magazine, as I was.

A new range would come out from a favoured designer. If I was feeling positive about a potential pregnancy, I'd order several things in a larger size, hoping to need it when the season arrived. When the hope was dashed, I'd ring up in defeat and revert to my usual size 10. Or the reverse would happen, and I'd order things small, tempting fate that I'd have to change and re-order them larger. So every aspect of life is affected, from the major to the minor.

Coping with Physical Invasion

Vaginal ultrasounds

Of all the techniques used within fertility treatment, vaginal ultrasounds seem to get the most negative comments from women. From Northern England to Northern Queensland, they seem to be the major source of embarrassment. Perhaps it is because these scans haven't been explained properly, as many women interviewed seem to react in shock that they were going to be scanned via the vagina. The more conventional ultrasound scan on the abdomen with a bursting bladder has been around for many years. The full bladder is necessary to push the uterus into a better viewing position. Maybe if the first time women were to have a vaginal ultrasound they knew what to expect, they wouldn't react with such embarrassment.

I had one recently to check my fibroids. I had been expecting a traditional scan, and then the doctor conducting the scan asked me to go to the loo (always a relief when having an external ultrasound) and she would continue the test with a vaginal scan. Having listened to the comments during interviews for this book, I wasn't sure what to expect. But the female doctor was great, the probe was introduced gently and it wasn't in the least uncomfortable, and I was sent off to the loo afterwards with some tissues to wipe away the gel used on the scanner.

So perhaps, as patients, we have to ask what kind of a scan we are to have, so we know what to expect and it subsequently doesn't cause embarrassment. I found it a great improvement on the bursting bladder scans, which are especially uncomfortable in early pregnancy. However, I do believe I would have been affronted if the scanner had been clad in the thumb of a surgical glove, with the other fingers dangling out, as has happened to many women:

> *Most of the treatments were reasonably well explained except for the internal ultrasound. It didn't occur to me that they could be done like that. I must admit that the older I became the more upsetting the vaginal ultrasounds became for me. I especially didn't like the use of a finger from a rubber glove as a protective sheath, the other fingers hanging down used to look really off to me. I used to wonder why couldn't someone make a sheath like a condom (without spermicide, obviously) to give the process a little more dignity.*

Another added: 'It's a bit like having protected sex.' An English patient commented:

> *I was sitting behind the screen on a fairly high bench when the doctor arrived to give me my first scan. I didn't really know what to expect. The next few seconds count as about the funniest of all my experiences. First of all, what I took to be the scanner was covered by just one finger of a polythene glove. The finger was then coated by a blue gel, which after much squeezing emerged reluctantly from a plastic bottle with a loud squelch, the kind guaranteed to have a classroom in uproar for 10 minutes (I am a teacher). While these preparations were going on, I assessed the situation and worked out what was going to go where judging by the shape of the scanner and the position the doctor wanted to put me in. At the same time I remembered the period-inducing pill I had taken, which had reliably produced a result that morning and realised the doctor wasn't going to get far with the scanner at all. 'Hang on a minute, I'll have to remove my tampon first.' He shot off behind the screen then asked with some concern if I had a replacement. It*

was an odd and slightly uncomfortable experience and I probably wriggled round a bit. When I was dressed and he joined me he said, 'I'm sorry, I didn't meant to hurt you.' 'You didn't,' I replied, wriggling slightly as I remembered the sensation. 'It's just that I don't think I would ever get used to it.'

Others mentioned the same surprise, even shock, indicating that they hadn't been told that they were to have vaginal scan. Only the word 'scan' had been used, so they assumed it was the traditional one on the abdomen. Doctors and clinic staff are so familiar with the processes that perhaps they sometimes underestimate the effect it will have on patients, some of whom have had very few internal examinations in their lives until now. Some women, like American writer Anne Taylor Fleming, in an article adapted from her book *Motherhood Deferred: A Woman's Journey* (GP Putnam's Sons, 1994), take a matter-of-fact approach to the vaginal scan:

I go into the examining room, strip from the waist down and take my place in the stirrups. The doctor appears. Boyish and solicitous, his hair beginning to gray like that of many of his patients, he is perfectly cast for his role as procreative assistant to a bunch of desperate women. Gently he inserts the dildo-like scanner and voilà, my ovaries appear as if by magic on the grainy screen. The doctor and I count together: One, two, three on the left side; one, two on the right [egg-producing follicles]. 'You have the ovaries of a 25-year-old,' he says, reaching for the syringe of my husband's sperm, now washed and sorted and counted. And with one deft whoosh through a thin catheter inserted up through my vagina and cervix, the sperm are sent spinning into my uterus.

The final word: 'It isn't particularly pleasant, the whole procedure, but you persist if you want to have a baby.' And of the older scans:

I remember when we had to go to the clinic in Brisbane and it was an hour and a half drive. At that time we had the old-fashioned ultrasounds where you had to have a full bladder, drinking gallons of water an hour beforehand. I think I knew every bump in the road to Brisbane.

Embryo replacement

As many infertility clinics are attached to teaching hospitals, quite often there are trainee staff present during treatments. Also, several specialist staff have to be there. Many women find this stressful. Again, because it is a regular occurrence for doctors, scientists and clinic staff, they can sometimes forget the dehumanising effect, as they try to get everything technically perfect. A woman from Australia's Gold Coast described her reaction: 'The last time I had a transfer they were all standing round the table and I was lying there naked, and I said if it's good enough for me to be lying here showing all, it's good enough for you, too.'

And another: 'I found it a bit embarrassing, when I went in to have the embryos put back. You have two or three nurses in the room, the doctor and the scientist and you are lying there with your legs open, it's quite humiliating.'

A patient from Northern England had a different perspective: 'I didn't care how clinical the experience was. I was 45 and we knew we had only one chance, the clinic had offered us that, and we were using donor sperm and donor egg to increase our chances. When our pregnancy test was positive, I couldn't have been more shocked if it had come out of the blue.' Carolyn, the nurse from Victoria, Australia, who described her IVF experiences in the previous chapter commented:

Now I am 17 weeks pregnant and a normal obstetrics patient, I find it hard to remember the embarrassment and discomfort. My husband and I feel so thankful and privileged that we conceived, and are well on our way to having our family. I think of the distant future when hopefully this baby is old enough, and if we can, I'd go through it again to have another.

Weight gain

In their efforts to do everything possible to maximise their chances of success, many patients go on a health kick during their attempts, and are specially careful about weight gain as the drugs used to stimulate the follicles can make some people bloated. Many people try to control excessive weight gain on their own. Others, like the following woman, seek help from a professional:

As I became involved with each IVF attempt, I went on a health kick. With the IVF drugs I put on excess weight. I then read about some studies in Adelaide which were proving that overweight women were finding it harder to fall pregnant than those at their normal body weight. So I employed the services of a dietitian to help me regain my normal weight. With her help and guidance, I was able to regain my normal weight. I was still seeing my dietitian with whom I had an appointment twelve days after my last transfer of frozen embryos. She suggested I seek help of a psychological kind and begged me to see the clinic psychologist. I found it amazing that someone treating me for weight loss recognised my emotional state and the clinic didn't.

Another, at the start of treatment, expresses her fear: 'I haven't started yet, but I am a bit worried as they all say the drugs make you gain a lot of weight. Will I look like a blimp? Will everyone know I'm having some kind of treatment?'

Mood swings

As if being infertile isn't enough to turn us into a neurotic mess, sometimes the drugs contribute to these mood swings. Both your natural psychological state and the drug-induced one should be carefully watched by you, your partner and the clinic.

The following comments voice a range of complex emotions:

'My failure to ovulate made me feel like a borderline fertility patient. Because I still had infrequent periods, there was always the possibility that we would do it on our own. The Clomid [clomiphene, a drug to induce ovulation] turned me into a hateful person, and as no other treatment was offered for many years, we focused on that other treatment, lots of holidays, using the time for us, completing a degree, and concentrating on careers and lifestyle.'

'The first time treatment failed, I felt horrible. My husband and I didn't leave the house for weeks,' said another. 'The hardest part was telling other people that we'd failed. The second time I was very, very angry — angry with myself, my husband and everyone around us. I wasn't nice to live with. In fact, I think I was the most horrible person I've met in my life.'

'I was having Clomid to help regulate my cycles and pretty soon the depression and mood swings kicked in. I had good days when I was invincible and bad days when I'd just cry,' said a Sydney woman.

'I found it stressful, I wasn't cranky, just stressed. I felt Alex didn't understand what I was going through. I think maybe I felt guilty, too, because I was the one with the problem. I did explain to him that if he wanted to leave me and have children with someone else he should — that's not what either of us wanted, but I felt he's got the right, if he wants children and I can't produce them. I'll never forget driving back from our first IVF attempt at Townsville and I said "That's the hardest thing I've ever done," and he said, "It's not hard," and at that point I just shut my mouth and didn't say any more. I thought he's got no idea what I've been through,' added a woman from Cairns.

Working around Treatments

Working during treatment cycles is complicated on many levels. There are the logistics of getting to the clinic or lab or surgery at the right time. Blood tests are usually carried out early in the mornings so clinics can get the results processed during the day and act on those results later in the day if necessary. These are usually done on a first-come, first-served basis and if you have to travel a long distance from home to clinic then to work, obviously the stress levels rise if the person in front of you has a long appointment and you are rushing. If you are involved in egg pick-up and transfer, you cannot really plan your days off until your period arrives, and even then it is up to the fine-tuning dictated by the drugs and the way your body responds to them.

If you plan to keep the whole thing a secret from your employers and colleagues, juggling this hidden agenda can increase stress levels. But if you do tell them, as I found

I had to, then you are aware of being watched, and regarded, from then on, as a much more temporary staff member.

This was the aspect I found most unfair. If you are trying to conceive normally, it is something very private, and you really don't have to say a word until you have a small tummy. No one is looking over your shoulder, looking for a replacement for you, while you try to conceive.

On a more profound level, the journey through fertility treatment touches areas of you that have never been explored — physically and emotionally — and they are of such significance that often the day-to-day happenings at work do seem very unimportant.

All journalists love gossip, and large publishing empires are a wonderfully rich source, but for the duration of my fertility treatment, I found it supremely uninteresting. Focusing on my work was still fine, producing a magazine is ever absorbing. However, for the first time in my life as a journalist, the periphery became non-existent.

The day-to-day monitoring of hormone levels, then the fourteen-day wait after treatment, are still about the only things I remember during that time. And the only relationships which seemed to matter were with my partner and the nursing sisters at the clinic.

As assisted fertility is still a relatively new field, employers have no guidelines on how to deal with it. It is not a spontaneous illness, yet it is something that requires medical intervention. In the ever-tight employment market and as someone who was responsible for a staff of people, I know how annoying it is to have someone *unreliable* who takes days off at a critical time. However, as a female boss I also found it much better when a staff member came to me and explained any problem they were having, as they did. You could then at least empathise with their difficulty, offer support when they needed it and also manage the office knowing there were times when that person would be away from their desk. It all depends on the attitude of the employer, your particular job and the way you and your partner have agreed to manage your treatment cycles.

There is no easy answer, but the following are some of the experiences of others in dealing with this complex issue.

Time off from work for me was hard initially because we kept everything a secret, which was the worst thing we could do. Now I've told them it really makes a difference. My boss was so supportive. She was on her way to a meeting interstate when I told her I was going into theatre for egg recovery in two days time. She told me to ring her and let her know what had happened. She rang me first to ask how it went and that was great.

_ℓ_

My boss told me not to worry about a thing, and said he'd already asked for someone to fill in for me. When I got to the clinic there were a couple of girls ahead of me and I panicked and knew I was going to be late. But because I'd told my boss, he knew where I was and there wasn't a problem.

_ℓ_

I am a nurse, and I work from 7 a.m. till 3 p.m. four days a week. So if I'm not there in the morning, I may as well not be there the whole day. I had to tell my immediate superior, who I consider a friend, because I thought I may become a little emotional. She asked me to tell the Director of Nursing because I work in a reasonably small hospital and my absence would have been noticed. My immediate superior was wonderful, saying yes, go for it, try and tell me as soon as you know when you will be absent. The director was much less so. I told her I was going on to IVF treatment and would need some time off. I said I realised it was disruptive and I would try and tell her the dates as soon as possible. Her response was that she'd worked with people before who had done this and they'd done it in their own time. I reminded her I couldn't tell precisely when my period would come and when things were going to start happening. She should have known you can't exactly organise your days off six weeks ahead. I told her that infertility was a medical condition and if I had appendicitis I'd have to ring and say I'd be off work tomorrow. As I had infertility, I could perhaps give her a few days notice, so she should be grateful for that, thank you very much. I think she was quite astonished by my response and has just kept her mouth shut since then.

<hr />

For work, I just said I had a hospital appointment. I'm a teacher and three of the seven visits to the clinic came in school holidays. The other four were split by a holiday so were less obvious. The clinic was about an hour's drive from the school. After I got pregnant, the head teacher asked me if that's what the hospital visit was about, but I was chicken and said no.

<hr />

As far as work is concerned, I am very lucky. I have an understanding boss and colleagues who would move heaven and earth for me if they could. My husband is not so lucky, but as he's a building surveyor, he does site visits which can be timed around scan and injection times.

Career Stalling

Because I so arrogantly assumed I could have everything, I didn't put my career on the back burner while I embarked on my quest for a baby. In many ways, it was a salvation, going into the office each morning to a demanding, stimulating job and an amusing and talented staff. No matter what the problems, after ten minutes in the office, most other parts of my life were blocked out by the demands of the magazine. I'd also seen my publishing 'mother' refuse a wonderful promotion because she was pregnant, then she had a miscarriage. By refusing that promotion, the course of her life changed forever, as did that of the magazine she was asked to edit at that critical moment. I was sure that was not going to happen to me.

Others, however, have refused promotions or unconsciously or consciously limited their career horizons as they tried to have a baby. They tell of their choices:

After 12 years of marriage we infrequently get asked if we plan to have a family. One day I overheard my brother telling someone that I didn't want children because I was a career woman. Comments such as these cut like a knife. In fact, I believe my career has suffered because I have not been as ambitious as I probably should be, always thinking that it was not worth applying for a particular promotion because I might be pregnant after that next treatment cycle.

~

I was a flight attendant and I grounded myself to work in an educational role, so I could work around my treatment. This work resulted in a move to the marketing department — then it was kind of mixing working and life around infertility treatment. I loved the marketing job. It was a great job, but it was much more stressful and I made the decision to leave. I'm the kind of person who is black or white — totally involved or not at all. I was very involved in that job, but made the decision to leave. I took a less challenging job locally to be near the treatment centre, and that was difficult: a different working environment, not so dynamic. Finances were difficult, as I was the main breadwinner. I was earning a good salary, then I cut that in half when I left.

Waiting To See If 'It' Worked

Almost every woman wanting a child, whether or not she has treatment, finds the fourteen days after she hoped to conceive, but before she can have a pregnancy test, the longest and most difficult days of her life. In the second half of the month, I would stop drinking alcohol, coffee and tea (wondering about the effects of caffeine), and take no drugs at all, even though I probably needed a strong tranquilliser. I would also organise my work life so I didn't take plane trips, even if there was an interstate meeting, as I'd read that pressurised cabins added to miscarriage risk in female flight attendants. It all would have sounded neurotic to my doctor or my friends, so I just quietly organised myself and said little. Only my beloved secretary of ten years sensed and would ask carefully if I wanted real tea or 'funny' (herbal) tea.

I can now read rationally the things the doctors say about behaving as normally as possible, but then, I was simply determined if anything carried a minuscule risk, I wasn't going to take it.

The investment after fertility treatment is immense. So many people have worked with you; you may have taken a lot of drugs and had many tests and bodily invasions. Has conception happened? Everyone agrees these days are torture. The medical staff empathise.

No one I interviewed found an easy solution. Perhaps this knowledge is the only solace. These days are pure hell for everyone, as the following comments reveal:

On the freeway heading home, I am already beginning the 14-day countdown to the pregnancy test — am I, am I not; am I, am I not — a moment by moment

monitoring, an imaginary ear to the womb intent on picking up any uterine sign of life.
Anne Taylor Fleming, *Motherhood Deferred: A Woman's Journey*, GP Putnam's Sons, 1994

～

I never found an easy way to deal with these days. I must admit I never thought the treatments would work, so I just thought of those days as a break before facing a week of having my period.

～

I think it's the worst 14 days of your life, that's all you think about. Everything physical or emotional is exaggerated. I used to go to the library every day and read the same books about pregnancy symptoms. Of course, I knew what the symptoms were, I'd read them so many times.

～

I pretended I was pregnant, pretended I couldn't stand the smell of some foods, felt nauseated, felt tired (good excuse for a nap), felt lethargic (who isn't after treatment?).

～

I found myself standing in the post office poking my boobs to see if they were really sore and swollen. People must have wondered what I was doing.

～

I remember waking up at 2 o'clock in the morning on the day my period was due and thinking bugger it, I can't wait another minute. I broke open the pregnancy testing kit and did the test, then woke my husband at 3 a.m. screaming out, 'I'm pregnant, I'm pregnant.'

～

We were becoming increasingly despondent about our DI attempts failing and booked a holiday. During our last attempt, which I only agreed to because of my husband, I did everything I was told not to do. I climbed ladders, went cycling, hoovered and generally treated it as an academic exercise. We got the fright of our lives when I found I was pregnant, we were absolutely ecstatic.

～

Talking about things falling out, I remember when I was in hospital having a transfer and we were all told to lie still for six hours afterwards. There was this girl lying in bed stiff as a board and there was a male nurse and he came in and said, 'Darling, what's wrong.' And she told him she wasn't going to move or even breathe. He asked, 'Why ever not?' and she told him her embryos were going to fall out. He said, 'Well darling, you should breathe.' They used to give you a medicinal brandy and you had a straw and he said, 'Would you like your brandy?' And she had it, but still remained there for six hours stiff like that. We were all killing ourselves laughing because when she got out of bed she was walking as though she thought these embryos were going to come out plop, plop, plop. I wonder how she managed the next fourteen days?

～

Both times I fell pregnant, I felt sick right from the start, the day after I conceived.

~ev~

During those fourteen days I could actually bear to walk through the babywear departments and dream; at other times, I did everything to avoid those places.

~ev~

Because I knew the drop in temperature meant my period would arrive the next day, I found myself taking my temperature earlier and earlier. I think 2 a.m. was probably the earliest. Then I would take it again a couple of hours later, hoping, if it had dropped, it was wrong. Only if it stayed in a high, straight line did I have any hope that I might be pregnant.

Dealing with Unsuccessful Treatments

We are all told the statistics for our particular treatments, but of course we all think we will be the special one to conceive first time. In my first cycle, which was really like a tracking cycle with inseminations, my progesterone levels were very high. The clinic sister told me quietly that only very lucky patients were pregnant first time, and she thought I may be one of them. I wasn't, but I didn't feel very worried as now we were having treatment I felt each month was positive, that at least there was a chance.

It is bewildering to know that even if everything is happening at exactly the right moment in a cycle with good eggs and sperm, that still you don't get pregnant each time. We all look for reasons why, but the experts say there is really no reason, it's just that humans don't conceive every time they are technically able, unlike other mammals.

We all continue to rack our brains for reasons, however, and drive ourselves crazy with 'What if ...?' Others explain their reactions to cycles which haven't worked:

To be honest, I really expected it to work the first time. I just thought it would be a case of me being given the right sperm. I couldn't believe it when I didn't become pregnant; every month I was convinced I was. I was probably imagining feeling sick and that sort of thing. We had the figures on the success rate from the hospital and the others, but you always think you're going to be the quick one.

~ev~

I found during the times between IVF cycles I couldn't stand it at work when women would come in with their babies. Sometimes I'd have to walk away, I couldn't serve them.

~ev~

I had a customer come in the other day, and we had seen her all during her pregnancy and now she had her baby. This woman actually said, 'Well, I've had her and I like her, but I'm not really fussed. I'm never having any more.' I actually couldn't speak, I can still hear her, and there she was with this beautiful four-week-old daughter, I could have ripped her away.

~ev~

The first time I went through IVF, I thought that's it. I didn't know much about the program and there wasn't a local support group. When I didn't fall pregnant, boy, was I a mess. The second or third time were not as bad, I think I was prepared.

The male perspective is very different, for apart from producing their sperm sample at the right time, they are largely left out of the physical processes, unless they administer the injections to their partner. One man commented:

I felt very involved and I was very disappointed when it failed. After the initial disappointment, each successive cycle I stood back a bit, a bit detached. Like everyone, the first time we thought yes, it will happen. When it doesn't, you come down flying down at such a great rate of knots. And I thought hang on a minute, we'll sit back and look at this. Each time the barrier gets stronger, even if you are rooting for it to work, you hold in a bit. After the first time I haven't let my emotions run away.

His partner added: 'You do that with the bills, too.'
Another male perspective:

Initially I felt tremendous excitement, I used to go along with my wife for the morning jabs and I just felt I wanted to be involved lock, stock and barrel, before I even went to work. I used to go in there in the morning and mostly just the wives were there and you do feel a bit of a lame duck in the waiting room, being the only guy there. But I felt I wanted to be there wholeheartedly. After we had our daughter, the second time round I felt I was getting a bit old and if it worked, great, if not ...'

His wife added: 'Yes, I knew even though you were in the room with me, you were no longer really there.' This need to impose some emotional distance is by no means unique:

My husband would become very involved then back off a little when it became too emotional for him. The consistent early mornings to get to the clinic were tough. Most of the time he was great and unselfish in his support of me as the one physically going through the treatments. I must admit I never thought the treatments would work.

NOT COPING

Not every story has a happy ending. One woman, Bronwyn, tells movingly of her struggle and her eventual decision to cease treatment.

'After living with my husband for nearly twelve years, we decided to marry in 1992. It was after much discussion that we decided we'd like to start a family.

'My husband, having been through the Vietnam War, had decided to have a vasectomy on his return from the war, after hearing and reading stories of horror in which children were born with severe illness and disabilities. Neither of us was sorry for this decision, although my husband now thinks it is the worst decision he ever made. We knew we had a problem up front as we confronted our specialist, who informed us that for Bill to have his vasectomy reversed would put him through much discomfort, so it was agreed we would try donor insemination, and if I was OK, we were told by our good doctor I would have a pregnancy in four months.

'Each morning I rose early and drove to the clinic for a blood test to check my hormone levels and finally the big day came; we were both excited. We waited two weeks hoping we'd be lucky, sadly we were not. Well, after six months of failures and six IUI [intra-uterine insemination] attempts, buckets of tears and hours of anger and frustration and the query of WHY still looming over us, we went back to our good doctor who suggested an investigation was called for. My dye test said I was OK, so everyone was baffled at why I'd not conceived.

'Realising then IVF was my only chance to have a family, I channelled all my energy into being positive at each attempt, fully knowing I was taking a gamble, the odds not being in my favour. I knew I had a 30 per cent chance — obviously the other side of that was a 70 per cent failure rate.

'Our next attempt was an IVF-related one with GIFT. I'm not my best in the wee hours of the morning, but I'd drive every morning to the clinic for my injections and blood tests — I so badly wanted our baby, I'd get up at 5 a.m. Somehow it doesn't seem fair. We persevered and ten days later found I'd produced twenty-three eggs and was in danger of hyperstimulation. Bill drove me to the hospital and blood tests from the night before revealed hormone levels too high to risk transfers.

'So my doctor did an egg collection (sounds a bit like a poultry farm) and the final count was sixteen — Wow! — out of the sixteen, only two fertilised! NOT A GOOD RESULT! I'm either stupid or just determined, I wanted our baby so badly, I went back again a few months later.

'More early mornings, more blood tests, more scans and after last time I was like a cat on hot bricks. At last we reached theatre day and we got the whole procedure this time — yippee! We had seven healthy eggs and three were replaced into the tube with the sperm. Three of the remaining four fertilised in the lab. Three needles later and fourteen days after theatre I get my result — negative.

'That was four GIFT cycles ago. And it's been about the same each time — good eggs, good sperm, good fertilisation, but no pregnancy. After this, I began questioning my doctor about fibroids and if they could be causing the problem.

'After consulting other specialists, the doctor decided to remove them and we set a date. Major surgery, and the worst of this was that I couldn't go through a cycle for three months. That three months went by fairly quickly and I started GIFT again. After this I felt positive and that all our troubles would be over.

'With a mixture of excitement and fear, I started early morning clinic visits again, more needles and blood tests, more scans. I responded well to the drugs and even after a long break, when theatre day arrived we collected fourteen eggs. I had my fingers, arms and legs crossed.

'I decided to donate nine to someone else if it worked. I had to phone the clinic lab to see how many fertilised. Only three out of eleven — my spirits plummeted. Three needles and two blood tests later, I got my result — negative again. I think this is the worst I've felt — I went into a deep depression and wondered if it was all worthwhile.

'Well that was my fifth attempt, and I then had only one super-ovulated cycle to go on Medicare. As I had some embryos frozen, I decided to do a frozen cycle. This would be the second time I'd attempted a frozen cycle and to be honest I wasn't looking forward to it.

'Even though I wasn't having injections, I still had to go to the clinic every day for blood tests to monitor hormone levels.

'I found I was at the clinic by day and the Emergency Centre at the local hospital at night for blood tests. Eventually the day and time for transfer arrived and I was back in theatre. Once the transfer is complete you have to lie still for four hours — it is the longest four hours ever. I can't sit still for five minutes, let alone four hours. We waited another two weeks for the result again — negative.

'Once again I dipped into the depths of depression. I should mention when I had the frozen transfer, of the four embryos thawed, only one survived. But then one is all you need! That cliche again.

'I went back to the specialist and after much discussion it was decided another investigation was needed — called a falloposcopy — which enabled them to look inside the tubes.

'I went into theatre hoping all our efforts were purely bad luck — my result was the worst possible news — one of my tubes was flat, stuck together, the other was full of adhesions. I was no longer a candidate for GIFT, but one for full IVF.

'Failure was never on my mind during my attempts. As my problem was purely and simply physical, I felt I'd be wasting time, positive energy and money on alternative therapy. After all, paying for Chinese acupuncture was not going to make my husband miraculously fertile.

'Owing to the IVF drugs, I put on a lot of weight and I employed the services of a dietitian to help me lose this weight. Over six months of hard work I regained my normal weight. I did this for my last Medicare rebated IVF attempt. I started this attempt on my husband's birthday.

'I started with the usual injections, had discussions with the doctor who insisted we double the hormone dose, despite my weight loss, and if all went to plan we would transfer four embryos and hope that at least one would implant. Due to the double dose of hormone I was extremely anxious and very concerned because of hyperstimulation. Our doctor explained we had to get as many eggs as possible despite the possibility of hyperstimulation, as this was my last Medicare-rebated attempt. We discussed how if my eggs didn't fertilise after two days they would be micro-injected — amazing the advances in a short period of time.

'The double dose of hormone worked and I had fourteen follicles. I went to theatre and was lucky enough to collect fourteen eggs. Out of these, eleven fertilised, which was very pleasing. After two days I was back to theatre again, in time to see our precious possibilities. I donned a mask and gown and wandered down to the lab to look down the microscope. Wow, what a fabulous sight, I had three four-cell embryos and one three-cell embryo. Then it was time for transfer, no anaesthetic. After the transfer, I was told to lie still for four hours. My remaining seven embryos were frozen. Two weeks, three injections and two blood tests later — I had my result, negative once more.

'At this point I went into shock, I felt dead, numb, and really just nothing. Determined as usual, onwards I plodded. Because I had seven remaining embryos frozen, I decide to straight away do a frozen cycle. No hormone injections this time, just a lot of blood tests — day and night. Once my levels were correct I was off to theatre, this time with a sedative to settle me down. Three out of four embryos survive the thaw.

'So I had them transferred. As the transfer was rather late, I decided to stay the night in hospital. No extra needles this time, just the blood tests.

'As I was still seeing my dietitian, I had an appointment with her twelve days after the transfer. She must have seen the future and suggested I seek help of a psychological kind — she felt I was borderline — whatever that means. She begged me to see the clinic psychologist. I admitted to myself I was not coping. I already knew the answer before I had my blood test. What I didn't know was how I'd cope with it — another negative result.

'This was a Wednesday. My appointment with the psychologist was on Saturday at midday, I realised at this point that this was far too late. By the appointment time my condition had deteriorated to such a state that I was admitted to hospital suffering from severe clinical depression. Before being admitted I had to go home and pack for hospital. I called in to work and told them I wouldn't be in for a while. I really don't know how I got home, everything was a great blur or haze. Depressed, I was very much so. I so desperately wanted out, I mean out permanently of this life.

'I began taking extremely large doses of paracetamol-type drugs, of course these didn't work. So deep was my depression, I felt so sad, so very alone, if I could have found a quick, certain way — a way that would produce a positive answer — to commit suicide, I would have.

'I continued to see the psychiatrist for some six months, then due to stress and prescribed anti-depressants, I found myself in the back of an ambulance, having suffered a major seizure. This placed me in hospital for eleven days. This suddenly explained why I'd had three car accidents and why I was at times strange. After my eleven days in hospital, I decided, with my husband's consent, to donate the three embryos I had in storage.

'Although this decision was a difficult one, it was made as I was sure I must never again see the door of an IVF clinic. It was also made not fully knowing how long embryos survived successfully in a frozen environment.

'Due to my continued illness, my marriage failed three months ago; my husband was unable to cope.

'IVF is not a quick fix for infertility — apart from time, money and good health, you need total commitment and support from your partner. I had none of this and it may have contributed to my failed sixteen IVF or related attempts. I so desperately wanted a child, I shouldered all the stresses associated with IVF.

'As I'd undergone four different programs I found they affected me differently.

'IUI I found embarrassing, success or not.

'GIFT I found sad and life-destroying, hard to explain really, but after each GIFT attempt failed I felt a little bit of me died.

'IVF was a combination of both GIFT and IUI. Frozen embryo transfers were difficult owing to the amount of blood tests, they were also embarrassing.

'I've been told I was obsessed and I'll swear I wasn't, nor am I now. I never looked at what I was doing as being obsessive, I believed in what I was doing, I believed in science, I believe in myself enough to believe what I was doing could lead to a successful pregnancy.

'My husband dutifully signed all the forms connected with IVF and related programs, at times he dropped me off at the hospital and at times picked me up, he most certainly wasn't involved except for these *duties*. And consequently all the stresses and pressures of IVF fell on me.

'Those last two weeks after transfer — I swear they are the longest two weeks of your life. I think of each attempt and as those fourteen days drew to a close, I usually could tell that I'd failed, though I lived in hope — after all, as patients of IVF, that is one thing we do a lot of.

'Coping so far with life without a child has been pure hell for me — my heart breaks every time I hear of an abused child or one being left somewhere. I hate living each day without my husband and the absence of a family that could have been.

'I've found through the media we patients of IVF are given a false impression of IVF. We are lead to believe this is a quick fix for infertility. It isn't. It takes time, money, patience and a hell of a lot of good luck.

'I don't have any regrets. IVF has taught me a great deal about life, and I do wish success for everyone else. I'm thankful we have IVF, and for the tremendously skilled medical and scientific people who make it possible.'

Chapter 8
Losing out

'My friend has a baby. It's four weeks old. I can't hold that baby. When she held it out to me, I told her it was tired and she should put it to bed. You're always the last to know that someone is pregnant. They find it very hard to tell you. It hurts that they don't tell you — but when they do, you feel jealous. There is no way I can congratulate someone who is pregnant.'

Within the crisis of infertility itself, there are many sensitive areas. Times when your head tells you one thing and your emotions behave in a contrary fashion. The two worst, in my view, are the pregnancies of people close to us, where you have to feign happiness, and indeed you do feel happy *for them*, but immensely sorry for yourself.

The second one is achieving a pregnancy which doesn't last. This is the worst crisis most of us will ever face.

Pregnancies of Others

The news that people close to us are pregnant brings with it many emotional overtones: pain, because you wish it was you; guilt, because you hate hating others who are successfully, joyously pregnant; resentment, because you can't see why it can be easy for others and not for you; and a combination of all of these things.

I'll never forget the night my closest colleague told me she was pregnant. I'd just had an early miscarriage and was still feeling empty and sad. We went to a business dinner and she refused the champagne that was offered, saying she was on a strict diet. She asked me if we could have coffee after the dinner and it was during this she told me that she was not drinking any more as she was pregnant. She told me with great sensitivity, even though I hadn't made a big thing out of my miscarriage. I was stunned and hastily said all the right things to her and headed home, feeling frozen inside.

This news was followed quite quickly by a similar, though less sensitive repeat broadcast from my other closest colleague. They were due at exactly the same time, and the timing couldn't have been worse — we were to have a major relaunch of the magazine that month. Fortunately, life was so busy it didn't give too much time to dwell on things, but as their tummies expanded, I felt huge pain as they came back from various doctors appointments and huddled together comparing their results. Because they were both close to me, I sewed pretty nighties for them and things for the babies, but in doing so I felt the mixed messages of wishing I was doing it for me and wondering if I was making this effort for them out of friendship or living vicariously.

87

We all survived, even the prams brought to the Christmas lunch. After my second miscarriage, another friend and colleague also conceived. I was hardened to it by now, but I was deeply, unreasonably angry with her for drinking and smoking her way through the pregnancy. I lectured her endlessly, trying to tell her how lucky she was and she shouldn't endanger this precious baby. But she was incapable of change, and had conceived so easily that she was very flippant about it all. Her pregnancy affected me more than the others.

Then following neatly on, my secretary became pregnant. She was rather different and more vulnerable, having had problems in the past, but again I felt unable to ask her many details or get involved in talking about the pregnancy. I was strictly business-like about it, it was the only way I could cope. I was so desperate that people shouldn't feel sorry for me that I was probably very remote with her.

I had had about two unsuccessful cycles of treatment when her baby was born. And because I had always been the person closest to her after her mother, she rang me from the labour ward, triumphant and happy. I truly hated her at that moment, no matter how fond I was normally. It made me feel that anything I had achieved professionally or personally were nothing, compared with this huge step into motherhood she had made, but which eluded me. I came off the telephone shattered. She wanted me to be proud of her, to have me say how well she had done delivering this fine, big baby so easily, and it was (unintentionally) the most cruel moment in my infertility experiences. When she had severe post-natal depression following this, I did feel guilty (again) for my initial reaction.

My feelings were also tempered by the knowledge that at the time my sister was desperately trying to conceive many years earlier, then suffering an early miscarriage, I was terminating an unwanted pregnancy. So I was aware of the peculiarity of fate.

We all react in different ways, but we do react, as the following people recount:

After investigations, we were basically told that my husband had no sperm, and that we had the choice of donor insemination or living without children — we were considered too old for adoption. I said I didn't want anyone's babies but Peter's, so we opted for the last solution — living without children and having lots of nice holidays, which we did for some years. But it really hit me that I still wanted a baby when my sister-in-law rang me up and said, 'I'm pregnant.' She was the one who had said she never wanted a baby.

With that couple childless, I thought I'm not the only one not to give my mum a grandchild. But at that moment, after she rang up, I thought I wish I could give my mum a grandchild, too. I just lay on the floor and cried my eyes out. I felt I couldn't say too much to Peter because we'd made a conscious decision we weren't going to do anything different to have a baby. But from that moment on, the feeling just got worse and worse. One Saturday morning we were lying in bed and I had to say something and I blurted out I want a baby, too, and it turned out Peter had been having the same feelings. We now have a wonderful little girl from donor sperm.

Lots of patients tell how they resent being left out when a close friend becomes pregnant — people simply avoid telling them, for fear of hurting them. Yet the omission is often worse. Like the following women:

Many of my friends have become pregnant in the past twelve months and they have felt terrible to tell me. Some of them put it off for months. One friend rang from the USA and began crying on the phone. When I asked what was the matter, she said I'm three months pregnant and I don't know how to tell you. I probably coped better than she did, because she was so devastated to tell me her good news.

I sometimes feel awful that there's a conspiracy in our group of friends, that everyone else knows, but you are on the outside. They don't know how to tell you, and I hate that.

Some, like this woman from Northern England, tell of the great care taken with them by family and friends:

After we found out my husband had no sperm, my sister announced she was pregnant. My world just fell apart. She and my brother-in-law were a great support to us, continually encouraging us to find a fertility clinic and seek treatment. During this time, I had good days, and bad days when I'd just cry. When our niece was born, her parents did everything they could to involve us, including ringing at 3 a.m. from the delivery room so we could hear the baby's first cries. They were wonderful. Another friend turned up on the night she was born with a huge bouquet of white lilies for us, knowing the mixed feelings we'd be having.

Others share their mixed experiences and emotions:

If friends became pregnant I used to get very angry and then I used to shut off and let the friendship slip away. If friends or family had a baby and I was expected to buy a present, I used to wait for a good day, race into a department store and put something on lay-by, and then get my husband to pick it up at the appropriate time and send it on. I went through a very bad time when my brother became an expectant father after a very casual encounter.

My husband insisted I see a psychologist after I shunned my family for their excitement over the pregnancy and a previous pregnancy of an unmarried sister. I saw the psychiatrist for three visits. He told me my anger was reasonable in light of my situation and this was the first time anyone had indicated to me that at least my emotions were normal.

Up to this point it had seemed they were just as irrational as the notion that trying to have a baby was difficult and a big deal. No one else among our family or friends had had the difficulties we faced. I remember asking him what would happen to all the bad feelings I had as a result of infertility if I was to have a baby. He said they would all fade and the intensity would go. I would still remember them, but I wouldn't live with them the rest of my life. I think that is when I decided to try harder for my family.

I felt jealous, wronged, isolated. Part of me hated her (my friend) and every other pregnant woman.

The week our doctor confirmed that we would have to have IVF to have our family, our closest friends came over to tell us they were unexpectedly pregnant for the first time. Knowing that she was expecting to have difficulty, it came as quite a shock. We were both very happy for them, but we were certainly not expecting them to get pregnant that quickly. I certainly found it hard to take at first, even though I wanted to act as though I was happy for my friend.

I had to work through it a bit; I did feel perhaps jealous, funny. I talked to my friend about it after a little time, knowing I shouldn't be feeling anything nasty — only I wished it was me. I thought to myself, Do I really want anything awful to happen to my friend or her baby? No way, I still want her to have a successful pregnancy, even if I can't. Throughout this year, a number of others have become pregnant as well, and fortunately no silly fool has said to us, 'When are you going to get pregnant?' — our close friends have helped guard us from that.

Pregnancy Loss

What is the hardest scenario for a fertility specialist? Most of the doctors I asked had the same response as Dr Steigrad, who said:

Telling a patient who is pregnant that she has a missed abortion — somebody who has struggled one way or another and they've had a positive pregnancy test and you send them off for an ultrasound and the scan says there is no embryo, or there is a sac and an embryo but no heartbeat — that's tough. When you think you've made it and suddenly it gets whipped away from you.

As everyone who has experienced this will tell you, it is one of those moments in your life when the world stops. Life will thereafter be measured as before or after that time. Having a miscarriage of a wanted baby is tragic to anyone. When you miscarry what you think may have been your only hope at having a baby, however, when you have gone to immense effort to get to that point, the feeling of desolation is overwhelming.

When I conceived it never occurred to me that anything would go wrong. A few days after finding out, however, my partner reacted badly to the news. My mother was in hospital having a mastectomy, and some slight bleeding began. Because my sister had experienced bleeding in all her pregnancies, but they had proceeded perfectly, I did what she had done and went to bed. Because my breasts were still puffed up, I still *felt* pregnant, and I hadn't lost any clots or anything, I was hopeful I'd be OK. Inevitably, however, heavier bleeding began and my gynaecologist ordered a scan.

The operator of the scanner explained that if you saw a pulsating dot on the screen, it would be the heartbeat and would mean all was well. It was obvious all wasn't well, there was no pulsating dot. I sat in the waiting area, mercifully a private spot kept I suppose for people in my position, and sniffed quietly, waiting for the radiographer's report. The pregnancy was not *viable* and my doctor booked me in for a D&C the following day, trying to be encouraging to me about next time. I am told hospitals try to organise things a little better these days, but then, when I woke up from the anaesthesia in my own room, I could hear bangs and thumps in the next room. Then I heard an enthusiastic lecture about natural childbirth. Oh, how I hated and envied those women in the room next door, and how I tried to go back to the blur of anaesthesia, anything to block out all the cheerfulness beside me.

Somehow I got home, blaming everyone for my loss. Now I can (just) accept that maybe it was a glitch of nature. When my doctor told me that statistically one in five or six pregnancies ended up this way, it didn't help. I was empty, felt a total failure, and was back to square one, not knowing if it would ever happen again. I felt more fragile than ever before.

About a year later, I got out the Clomid prescription and tried again. Miraculously, it worked, and this time my partner was great, we immediately took a relaxing holiday and came back to have a six-week scan. This time the radiographer saw two sacs — twins — I was over the moon. The scan hadn't showed any heartbeats, but no one seemed worried, it was very early and the sacs were the right size. I didn't tell anyone except close family as I was superstitious after the previous time.

At a pre-Christmas staff lunch, I was standing washing up and felt a suspicious dampness in my knickers. I went to the loo and there was an ominous pink stain. Full of dread, I got into bed and stayed there, hoping it would go away. This time it didn't become heavy bleeding, so I still hoped and my breasts were still sore, so I still *felt* pregnant. I bitterly regretted doing the big lunch as I felt all the work had triggered this. You have to blame something. I stayed in bed and my family and friends looked after me as my partner had to go away to work. After a couple of weeks, I felt my breasts starting to go down, though I prodded at them so often to see if they were still big and sore, they probably stayed that way longer than they should have. I kept taking my temperature and while it stayed high, it reassured me that the hormones were still holding up. I rang my gynaecologist and he suggested I have another scan, by now, the spines and heartbeats should be visible. A friend took me to the hospital, and I had a repeat of the previous time — only this time, I couldn't stop crying. I cried all the way home, phoned my partner in London and couldn't even tell him for sobs.

The same scenario, back to the hospital the next morning for a D&C. Blighted ova, the term chills my heart. Empty sacs. Empty me. I became a sleepwalker.

The publisher at the time called me down the day I went back to work and said, 'What are you doing here, you look terrifying, you look like a ghost.' And that is what I felt like. A part of me became numb. I lost the ability to cry. I became numb and stoic, and very little touched me. My gynaecologist suggested I talk to the counsellor attached to their fertility clinic, and then suggested we start serious investigations to have a successful pregnancy next time, which we fortunately did.

Having a plan, something to go forward with, helped me survive. But I certainly didn't take my son's eventual birth for granted until he was actually in my arms. I read all the books that told me when a foetus was viable so I didn't feel confident till after that 32-week stage.

In the two weeks before he was born, he stopped moving and I experienced a night of total devastation, worse than anything so far. I felt I'd gone that far and lost the baby again. The same numbness (which had relaxed slightly) returned. I felt I'd never have the baby I wanted so much. I'd have to start all over again.

No one could understand my despair, as I walked around with a huge tummy. My doctor must have sensed my fears, I couldn't really communicate the subtleties in French. However, he ordered foetal heart monitoring every few days until the birth, and nothing could have helped more than being strapped up to a machine and hearing the thump, thump, thump of the baby's heart and seeing it printed out on reams of paper.

Pregnancy loss is never easy, but if it is a pregnancy you've waited years for, worked hard for, the loss is worse than anything imaginable. Worse because you are losing a potential life, one you haven't had a chance to know, but want so badly. It is also difficult because it is a bereavement few people acknowledge. They make cliched, painful statements like 'It wasn't meant to be, you'll be fine next time.' And because you may have been pregnant only a couple of weeks, most people can't acknowledge how real it was to you — even your partner.

The following are other patients' experiences:

In our last cycle of DI, I was fed up and treated it a bit like an academic exercise. We got the fright of our lives when I found I was pregnant. We were absolutely ecstatic, we were going to be a mum and dad after all. Our happiness was short-lived. Our baby died, unbeknown to us, at nine weeks and I didn't miscarry until thirteen weeks. I don't need to say how this felt; suffice to say that day will stay with me forever, and still strikes my heart cold.

Our family and friends, with the exception of one, were wonderful, flowers arrived by the minute and we wandered around in a daze. It's still pretty much a black fog when I think back — it was about six weeks after this that I started remembering things again.

The one friend we lost was herself six months pregnant and wrote and told me it had probably happened for the best and better luck next time. Needless to say, I decided our friendship wasn't worth suffering such blatant ignorance. No one will ever know why our baby died, but so much good has come of him being round for such a short time and no one in our family will ever forget him. My sister and brother-in-law named a star for him.

◦—

Our first pregnancy ended in miscarriage at seven weeks and the second went to full term with our lovely little boy. During the first, brief pregnancy, we were in a state of shock that it had actually happened and it was over before we had actually come to terms with the idea of having conceived a baby. The second time we were both terrified during the whole pregnancy and unfortunately we tried not to worry each other so we didn't really confront our fears with each other until three days after Tim was born. As a result, the pregnancy was not as joyous as it should have been, but was clouded with apprehension and fear.

◦—

Our first IVF attempt went quite normally and we had prepared ourselves that it could go either way and pregnancies didn't normally happen first time round. But the pregnancy didn't last. Two days after my D&C we had an engagement party to go to — all our friends were going to be there, including friends who had just announced they were pregnant. I was feeling extremely BLAH and basically that night I cracked up. In retrospect, it probably wasn't a good idea to have gone. I certainly remember in those few weeks that was all I could think about and if someone asked me how I was who didn't know what I'd been through, I found it very difficult to answer that question.

◦—

You hear all sorts of stories about things going wrong: having problems conceiving in the first place, then asking yourself is it going to be all right from the word go. Maybe we get so filled with so many negatives that we don't think of anything positive. And that is a lot of our problem in life. When you're going through IVF, you think: How many eggs will I produce, how many of those eggs will fertilise and become embryos, and out of those embryos, how many are going to be normal? How many of these are going inside, and then are they going to implant? And you think, wow, I'm pregnant. Then I lost the baby. Everyone thinks once you're pregnant, you're home. It's not until you get to that stage at two months and you lose it, then you think OK, I'm going to try again. OK, I'm going to go through that whole cycle again, then I'm going to lose it. Am I going to lose it at two months, at three, five seven or nine? When you start IVF, all you're worried about is conceiving a child, you don't worry about those nine months afterwards, or about miscarrying. When it happens next time for me it will be a huge obstacle.

◦—

A friend of mine has been pregnant three times with IVF and miscarried three times. It's devastating. To actually get the word that you're pregnant is a coup.

◦—

I went in and had a blood test and the clinic rang up and said we've got a problem. We don't know whether you're pregnant or not. I have two tests on your blood that are positive and one that is not confirmed. I had to come back in three days time. So you get through that and you are ecstatic and everything is rosy, though they even say in the brochures you can have a positive pregnancy test and a pregnancy may not eventuate. I was told 'You're sorta pregnant.' What's 'sorta pregnant'? It's horrible. They said on a scale of ten, you are a six. What does that mean? The stress that causes is so high. They classed it that I was pregnant for a full week. I asked how do you buy clothes for a sorta baby?

~ ❧ ~

I was really lucky. I had had one early miscarriage and was now pregnant for the second time. I was in a fairly fragile emotional state, recovering from being attacked and robbed some months earlier, so was also under the care of a psychiatrist. I started to bleed, and went to my new young gynaecologist. He immediately gave me two injections of progesterone. He said he wouldn't wait for test results to come in, that he would give me the progesterone immediately, as it wouldn't hurt me or the baby if I didn't need it. He was in touch with my psychiatrist and very aware of how important this baby was to my emotional healing. It turned out my levels were very low and I did need the progesterone, and now my lovely son is three years old.

~ ❧ ~

After two early miscarriages, I was successfully pregnant, with the help of the fertility clinic in timing things, and Clomid to make me ovulate properly. I was sent for a scan at eighteen weeks and was devastated to find there was a major problem with the development of the baby and I had to go into hospital and have labour induced. As I was going through this awful labour, all I could think of was how soon could I try again, and even if the problem was genetic, I'd take the one-in-four risk. For weeks afterwards, I would burst into tears in the middle of the street. To make matters worse, my partner and I had a huge fight about the baby the night before the ultrasound, so he feels terribly guilty now.

Chapter 9

Artificial Insemination—With Partner or Donor Sperm

Question: Why were men designed in such
a way that it takes 600 000 sperm to fertilise one egg?
Answer: Because they are men and won't stop to ask directions.
**From *The Donor Conception Support
Group Newsletter*, Sydney, 1997**

Artificial insemination is assisted reproduction in a simpler form than IVF, with no surgical procedures needed. It usually involves no more than prepared sperm from the partner or fertile sperm from a selected donor being inserted into the woman's vagina during her fertile days of the month. The sperm is introduced via a tiny plastic tube and a speculum — rather like having a cervical smear test.

This is for *male factor* infertility, where the woman's tubes and uterus show no abnormalities, but the semen analysis has indicated problems — major or minor — with the sperm.

There are three abbreviations you need to be familiar with in treatment using artificial insemination. They are:

- **DI** or **donor insemination**, where the semen that is introduced into the cervix comes from a selected donor. This procedure used to be call AID (artificial insemination donor), but this latter acronym was dropped with the advent of AIDS;
- **AIH** or **artificial insemination** using the semen of the husband or partner. Frequently, this is used when the partner has a poor sperm count, but doctors feel they can process the semen to get a better quality sample, with more chance of fertilisation. This is also the method used if there is a problem in the male preventing normal intercourse;
- **IUI** or **intra-uterine insemination**, which is sometimes used if the quality of the woman's cervical mucus doesn't allow sperm penetration or simply to give the sperm a better chance to reach the ovary, with less obstacles to pass. This technique is used for both DI and AIH.

Not many men have no sperm at all, the condition known as *azoospermia*. However, an increasing number of men have lower counts than required for a successful conception. The old cliche of 'One is all you need' is simply not true, except when using assisted reproductive technology.

The major breakthrough for *male factor* infertility in recent years has been the introduction of ICSI — a technique developed in Belgium, where eggs are stimulated and retrieved as with IVF treatment, then one sperm, even an immature one, can be injected into the centre of the egg and fertilisation can follow. The fertilised egg or eggs are replaced into the woman 48 to 72 hours later, as with IVF, and after fourteen days, tests will tell if implantation has occurred and a pregnancy has resulted. However, this treatment still requires all the IVF drug therapy for the woman, who may have perfect reproductive health herself, plus the time and dedication to attend egg pick-up and replacement, and the generally low success rates common in all IVF treatments.

If there is sufficient good-quality sperm in among the low-quality, lab technicians can process it to achieve a concentration of the best sample, to be inserted into the cervix or directly into the uterus of the woman. This can also be combined with egg stimulation to guarantee ovulation in the woman. 'We have a group of patients where there is no abnormality in the woman and a mild degree of male factor abnormality,' said Dr Stephen Steigrad, 'so we are combining ovarian hyperstimulation with intra-uterine insemination of processed sperm. And that is a halfway house to telling patients there is nothing that we can do for them, and the only thing we can do for them is IVF.'

If this kind of treatment or ICSI is not an option, then donor insemination, adoption, or living without children are the only remaining alternatives.

Donor insemination (DI) is in some ways the ugly duckling now in assisted reproductive techniques. It is less invasive and technically far simpler than its high-tech cousins, and as around 90 per cent of couples choose to keep their treatment a secret, there is not a lot of open discussion on the subject. The clinic or doctor select a donor based on similarities of race, physique, blood group and interests of the husband or partner. Also, as with artificial insemination from the husband, the woman's fertile time is established by blood tests, temperature charts, mucus quality or a home ovulation kit, and the sperm is introduced into the cervix on successive days in this fertile period.

The semen used in DI has been donated by screened donors, who have offered to assist childless couples. Historically, donors were medical students. This was at the time when fresh semen was used and the students were geographically available. Now they come from wider areas of society and are often men who have had their families and donate sperm prior to undergoing a vasectomy.

In countries with a background based on British law and customs, the sale of human gametes is usually considered unethical. Altruistic donation is the only source possible. A donor can receive a minimal amount for travel or other expenses incurred. In the United States, however, 'donation' is much more commercial and sperm 'donors' are paid a fee, depending on the clinic they attend. Unfortunately, this can lead to men concealing health problems in order to qualify. However, if the sperm is subsequently frozen and the man re-checked, as explained later, this should eliminate risks.

All donors are screened for hereditary diseases and complete a form to assess if they have been involved in at-risk-for-AIDS activities. The donor is checked for infectious diseases and a blood sample taken to assess his blood group. The semen is checked for its fertility potential and then sealed in straws, carefully coded, and stored in liquid nitrogen at minus 196°C. Storage at this temperature is possible for many months or years. The donor returns after six months and a second blood test is taken to ensure he was not in a window period for infection from HIV (pre-AIDS) or hepatitis B or C. It is only after this second blood test is clear that the stored semen is available for use.

When this time comes, the semen is thawed at room temperature for ten to fifteen minutes, and then a tiny drop is checked to see it has survived the thawing process. If so, the inseminations can proceed.

Often, talk about DI immediately stimulates titillating talk about people creating super-races — everyone seems to have seen a television program about the propagation of the mind of Einstein in the body of Sharon Stone. Or they have heard a story about a white woman giving birth to a black child or vice versa, via a sperm bank mishap. Or even worse, they know all about the subject via an intense interest in the cattle industry!

It is also strange that genetic *paternity* seems to have a more emotive connotation than, for example, if a sister or friend donate an egg, often seen as a loving, feminine act. If a brother or close friend volunteers his sperm, however, it is seen as a kind of dirty joke and reported thus.

Is it that the exchange of eggs is seen as a medical act, whereas the exchange of semen is seen only in its sexual context? This quote seemed to sum up the general community attitudes to DI:

Donor insemination is made up of two taboos — sexuality and reproduction. Both are intimate, making it difficult to discuss even in the 'nineties.
From *The Donor Conception Support Group Newsletter*, Sydney, May 1996

LEGAL ISSUES

There was a time when the 'social' father of a DI child had to adopt that child after its birth. Now, in most countries, the DI child has the protection of being legally regarded as the child of the partnership, with all the rights of natural children.

Before DI is carried out by a clinic, both partners must sign a consent form to protect all parties. In most cases, couples insert the male partner's name on the birth certificate.

For children born from donor eggs or donor embryos, laws have had to be constructed to clarify the meaning of mother and father in a licensed treatment. The legal mother of the child is the woman carrying and delivering the child and the legal father is normally the husband or partner of that woman.

This law, while clarifying the situation for couples with children from donor eggs or embryos, complicates it for couples wishing to have a child through surrogacy (see chapter 15). This is because, in terms of the law, the surrogate mother — not the commissioning mother — is the legal mother.

Establishing Ovulation Times

Whether your partner's sperm is being used, or that of a selected donor, the key to it all is the timing of the inseminations. At the time I was attending a clinic, ovulation timing for artificial insemination was established by blood tests, combined with assessment of mucus quality. These required early morning trips to the fertility clinic, followed by a telephone call to the clinic in the afternoon to see what was happening to the hormone levels and whether ovulation was imminent. Now, many patients are offered the use of home ovulation kits, which, if you live a long distance from the clinic or have a demanding morning schedule, save the stress of getting to the clinic early. Clinic staff report the same success rates with both techniques.

Temperature charts give the broad outline of the length of your cycles, and from this the clinic staff can work out when they should start monitoring you before ovulation happens. The first cycle of artificial insemination usually involves working out what is normal for your body and your hormonal state. The blood tests check for the surge of luteinizing hormone (LH) which precedes ovulation, and then the progesterone test about one week after ovulation was due confirms that ovulation has taken place.

In my first cycle, I was shattered when they told me they didn't think I'd ovulated successfully as my LH levels didn't go very high, then when they read the progesterone levels, they were high enough to indicate a pregnancy. When the doctor checked all the results at the end of the cycle, he suggested that I had what he termed a 'narrow fertility window' — that the LH surge had actually happened in the 24-hour period between the two blood tests. He suggested that if I had had another blood test in the evening, that would have shown the level for which they were looking.

When I look at the photograph of my mischievous eight-year-old above my desk, I wonder that I had so little faith that he would actually eventuate. In the clinic waiting room, you didn't do too much talking to others. You didn't really know what they were there for — whether it was for simply monitoring their cycles, for DI or AIH, or for any other fertility treatment. Most of us had to get out of there as quickly as possible and go to work, so the main preoccupation was your place in the queue. I do remember one morning there was a ripple of interest in someone's blood test; maybe she was pregnant, and I felt a pang of envy. I never saw her again, however, so I didn't discover the outcome.

Back in Sydney a couple of years ago, I called in to the clinic to say hello to the sister in charge and a morning coffee was in progress with the Donor Conception Support Group. I stayed and chatted for a while and heard some of their remarkable stories of surviving infertility.

While doing research for this book, I sat down for an evening with several couples from this group to learn of their particular experiences — from finding out about their husband's infertility, their experiences with various clinics, to their hopes and fears for their children. I also talked with the senior clinic sister, Eva Durna, about her experiences with donor issues in her twelve years of involvement with the fertility clinic at the Royal Hospital for Women in Randwick, NSW, Australia.

The Option of Donor Insemination

Sperm failure — finding out

Most fertility specialists in Australia now report that they test both partners simultaneously. This hasn't always been the case. It used to be that the man was often the last person tested, and then often as a final resort. If your doctor doesn't suggest testing you both thoroughly, change doctors or seek another opinion, as you can spend months of stress and heartbreak dealing with one problem, only to find the true difficulty is entirely unrelated.

The reason doctors now test both partners to get a complete overview before commencing treatment is that if they only test the sperm and that is defective, they may assume the woman is fine, and she may not be, or vice versa. If tests are carried out on both partners simultaneously, there is a sense of being united in the quest for a baby, and problems in either or both people are talked about as part of the overall treatment strategy, avoiding the blame factor for either partner.

One couple tells of years of testing on the woman before the husband, already a father, was tested:

'I knew I might have problems, we just hoped it [a pregnancy] would happen. We waited about a year before we went to see someone, but I was convinced it was my fault,' said Caroline.

'I already had two children from my first marriage,' adds her husband.

Caroline continued: 'I had CAT scans, blood tests galore and spent a year and a half on Clomid. Then I changed gynaecologists and when he put me into hospital to do a laparoscopy, he also tested my husband and found he had a major sperm problem. It's not unusual for that to happen — for the woman to have lots of tests and treatment before someone thinks to test the man. We were told together at the gynaecologist's office. Because he already had two children everyone thought he was fine, but sperm counts can change. At the same time, we were told our only option was DI or adoption, so I guess you think this is where I go next. You don't have any choice but thinking about the next step, which happens to a lot of people. You go from one step to another without getting any chance for things to sink in and for you to really think about it.'

'It's like being hit in the face with a brick,' said her husband.

A Sydney couple, Warren and Leonie, tell:

I don't think we'd been frantic about having a child, we just assumed a baby would come along after a while. Originally I had a test that said I had a low sperm count, but they didn't say it was nil or that the motility was low. At that time, my wife Leonie had an ovarian cyst removed, then we just left it to nature. We went overseas for six months and hoped.

His wife adds:

> *Yes, we made love under the Colosseum, all of that. We deliberately did it, and there was someone perving in our campervan window. That put a stop to that, I can tell you. We had fun trying. Eventually, we'd done everything: the Colosseum hadn't worked, I'd got a job, it hadn't worked, left work, took a year off work, it hadn't worked, we knew we needed help. About this time I bought a book about infertility by a woman gynaecologist and a lot of my questions were answered. We had a friend whose sister worked at a major hospital. She mentioned there was a fertility clinic there, so we made an appointment. We were both tested at the same time. Warren's semen had to go for a special test as it came back with a report that there was low motility. It took a couple of months to come back, telling us the tails were deformed and they weren't going to swim anywhere. That was a long couple of months. At that time [the early 1980s], there was a six-month waiting period. We took twelve months to decide whether or not we were going to have DI. Warren was ready to go, but I wasn't.*

He continues:

> *I was at work in the city the day I was told this and I just wandered round the city for a while, letting it sink in. It was a real shock. We came home that night and had a good cry about it. I actually left work, I couldn't stay there that day.*

A third couple tell of their experience with a urologist, who was reluctant to discuss the bad news with the husband. 'We had an indication a few years ago that Jeff might have a problem, so we thought about that straight away.' He adds:

> *It [infertility] was confirmed over the phone and the urologist didn't want to talk to me. He simply said there was a referral in the mail to go to a DI clinic, and he didn't want to talk with me further. I wanted to go in and see him and he wouldn't let me. So I went through the shock of it, denial, alone. It was very hard, he simply didn't know how to handle it. He was quite encouraging with the first test ... saying you know there is always IVF and all sorts of things, but at least you have got some sperm. So we'll just do these extra tests on you just to see the options. And that's when he decided there was no way IVF or anything else would work. Then he didn't want to have anything to do with us.*

'Then there was a three-month wait to get in to see the fertility clinic,' said his wife Michelle. 'In hindsight, it was good having this time, but then we didn't think it was good. We actually needed to see someone right away. We were floundering alone. They should have referred us to a counsellor or social worker, or somebody who knows something about it.'

A couple from the north of England tell:

Our first sperm test was poor so they suggested another one in three months. I went back for the results and they said the second test was nil also. I had to go home that night and tell my husband. Then they said they would do a biopsy to see if there was anything inside that they could put right. Because we were in England, we had to wait more months and time was going by and we were getting more and more uptight. They found baby sperm and wondered if they could stimulate them to grow. They put him on a fertility drug for four months and said if that didn't work, it wasn't going to work.

So we went back to the doctor and he said you have three options: (1) adoption, then he looked at our charts and said we were too old for that; (2) DI, but we didn't ask and he didn't explain further; and (3) we could forget about babies and have some nice holidays and think about it as a natural vasectomy. Which wasn't very pleasant really, looking back on it.

A man, already a father, commented on his vasectomy reversal:

We have no choice but donor sperm because since my vasectomy my body has been producing anti-sperm antibodies. I didn't realise that when you have had a vasectomy, sperm escape into the circulation.

The body hasn't met up with them before, as they were enclosed in the reproductive duct system up until the vasectomy. Your body reacts to them like it would to any foreign body, it makes anti-sperm antibodies and tries to kill them off. I am told the longer it is between having a vasectomy and having it reversed, the less chance there is of the reversal being satisfactory. But no one told me that when I went in for the original operation.

Starting treatment

Once couples have both been investigated, diagnosed and accepted on a donor insemination program, they then wait for communication from the clinic to tell them when the clinic has matched a donor, and when they can start. The clinic staff ask the date of the last period and the approximate length of cycles to calculate the correct day in the cycle for the first visit to the fertility clinic. In the first cycle, they will test hormone levels — particularly progesterone after ovulation — as well as taking blood or urine tests to determine ovulation.

Eva Durna, Senior Clinic Sister at the Royal Hospital for Women in Randwick, NSW, Australia, talked about the differing reactions of patients to this method of conception:

I think the most stressful time for patients is before they start treatment. The waiting time, making the huge decision whether they should or not embark on this big journey. It involves someone else's gamete [dictionary definition: sexual protoplasmic body or germ cell, which unites with another for reproduction]. *I would say the average time of grieving is six months, but then it's individual, it's different for everyone. We had a couple on the program last year — they started the year before that — and they knew about the husband's infertility for only two months and she was very keen to start. She pushed it through, but the husband wasn't ready. When she had the first insemination the husband came in, too, and he just couldn't cope. She didn't come back for the second insemination. They left it that month and went back for counselling. I had a couple of sessions here at the clinic with them, too. I could really feel his pain, I still can. So they discontinued treatment. She went back to the doctor, talked with the social worker and spent more time in here talking. And it took them about three months to decide to come back. She had four cycles and conceived, and now they have a lovely little girl. And he loves the baby.*

People share their experiences of treatment:

I was surprised when the doctor at the fertility clinic told me he was going to test me as well. At each level, I was sure they'd find something wrong and the dream of a baby would be snatched away again. At last all the tests were complete and we'd passed, me medically and we-the-couple psychologically when we saw the counsellor. Then I waited for a phone call from the clinic to tell me when I could start. A random call came in the middle of a busy afternoon and I discovered it was the clinic sister. A sweet, firm voice told me they had matched donors for us: there was a six-foot, grey-eyed unproven donor for the first three cycles as is their policy, and a six-foot three, hazel-eyed proven donor for the next three cycles. I promised to telephone at the start of my next cycle. There was an odd, surreal sense that you have been to the genetic supermarket. It is just a weird situation to be discussing. But it is not something I could talk about later with my husband, in case he saw my reaction as negative.

The sister told me they would take a blood sample each day to check when I'd ovulate, and a sample of mucus — a bit like a mini-smear test. As she finished, she told me I must ring at 4 p.m. every afternoon after the blood test to see if I was due to ovulate. She also explained that the first month is spent finding out the way your body works and its hormone levels and functions, so I would need a couple of other blood tests later in the cycle, to see if my progesterone level was high enough to hold a pregnancy.

'We don't always have to do blood tests now to determine ovulation,' said Eva Durna. 'The patients can choose to have either blood tests or home tests. You just have to urinate on a stick for ten seconds and read it, starting two days before you are due to ovulate. It is a very sophisticated test, very sensitive and very easy to read. It measures the luteinizing hormone in the urine, just as we can also measure it in the blood. Patients don't have to ring us, they just come in when the test indicates and have their inseminations done. And they have another insemination the next day. The pregnancy rates are the same as with the blood tests — and it saves time in travelling to the clinic, and blood tests are much more expensive.'

Patients add their comments:

'Home ovulation kits would have been a miracle for some of the women coming to the clinic. I remember one poor woman racing in from a factory job. She actually started work at 7 a.m. and had to come up to the clinic in her coffee break at 8 a.m., on the bus. She was so stressed each time, as a friend was covering for her, I wonder if she ever conceived.'

'It is better now there are more fertility clinics. One woman I talked to came from a remote country area and she would phone the clinic when her period began and then estimate a time to come down and stay at a motel in the city for her ovulation and inseminations. Invariably, the stress involved in packing, travelling and tests would delay her ovulation and instead of spending a few days in the city, she had to spend over a week. And the accommodation costs were very expensive.'

'I left home at 5.45 a.m. so I'd get there at 6.45, thinking I'd be the first one there,' said Leonie, who had to travel from an outer suburb to the city. 'Then I'd see three other women in front of me, and the pressure, the pressure I'd feel to get through and get out and get to work on time. I knew I'd have another hour there. The door didn't open till 7 a.m. and everyone knew who was first, no one pushed in.'

'At my clinic there was a board where you wrote your name,' said Michelle. 'One woman came in and put her name first on the board, before everyone else. There was a big argument in front of everyone with the clinic sister. The woman told the sister you said to put my name first on the board. The clinic sister said she told her the first thing she should do was put her name on the board.'

'You never offered to let anyone who was flustered go in before you. I made that mistake a couple of times, only to find they wanted to talk about something and were really ages,' added Michelle.

'By the third child I was waiting till after the early rush,' said Leonie. 'I'd arrive with a suitcase full of toys for my children to play with. That's another thing, if you already have a child it's hard to find someone to look after them at that time in the morning, also without explaining why you have to go out at that time. I used to feel guilty bringing the children, but then one time the clinic sister told me it was a positive thing, and it gives people hope.'

Treatment experiences

As with other forms of assisted conception, during treatment the fertility clinic is the centre of the universe, the place where all the answers are. The clinic staff know each subtle change in your reproductive system, and what's more, they seem to find it interesting — well, it is their job. Each month, ovulation is pinpointed and inseminations are done at the critical moment, and repeated the following day, unless there is a shortage of the sperm selected for you — as in some racial groups — when they can only *afford* to do one insemination because of a low supply of racially matching sperm.

'I felt a bit like I was attached to the clinic by an umbilical cord. All these intense experiences between me and my body were really only shared, or of interest to, the clinic. Even my husband couldn't get too excited about my LH levels or the state of my mucus,' said a Brisbane woman.

'Social activities were hard, too, like going away for a weekend,' said another. 'We came up from a weekend in the country for a special blood test. The girl I was staying with was an experienced laboratory attendant. She kept saying, why can't you have the test at the local hospital. And I had to lie. She knew something different was happening and she kept asking a lot of questions which made me quite irritated, specially when I came back with a really big bruise.'

'I suddenly started wearing long sleeves to hide the bruises in the crook of my arm so people didn't think I'd suddenly become a drug addict,' another observed.

'People would say how did you get a bruise there and I'd say I slammed it in a filing cabinet. I'm sure my mother thought I had a terminal illness I wasn't telling her about,' commented Michelle.

'I did feel a bit strange after the first insemination. Semen usually implies a really intimate act, and having it placed into my vagina, in a straw through the metallic apparatus of a speculum is hardly intimate. My thoughts did wander a bit the first time, lying on the couch in the cubicle for my twenty minutes,' revealed a Melbourne woman.

'My husband and I went for the inseminations together and afterwards I felt excited, relaxed and happy. A bit like we'd done something a bit naughty.'

'I used to rush down to the loo and put in my old diaphragm or a tampon, hoping to hold it all in there to add to my chances of conceiving,' said another. 'I felt really stupid at a lecture by the head doctor, when he patiently explained (others had the same idea) that our vaginas were not an open tube and that the vaginal walls spent most of their time folded against each other. I used to also wonder if I had an *orgasm afterwards it would help things along, too, but I didn't dare ask the doctor about that.'*

<hr>

'*My husband always came with me for the inseminations. He told his boss why he needed to be absent and there was never a problem. We didn't expect any problems and we didn't get any,' said Caroline.*

Julie, from York, England, tells of her moving experience:

My mother came with me on two occasions. The time our baby was conceived mum was there with me. She's quite proud of the fact that she was one of the very few mums actually present at her grand-daughter's conception. I asked her to hold my hand and send good vibes through for me. She's very psychic, my mum, she always seems to have the right vibes.

Waiting and expectations

'It is helpful for us for the patients to know as much as they can understand, and it is very important that they don't have high expectations that they are going to get pregnant quickly,' said clinic sister Eva Durna. 'You can usually sense how much information people can take in. People have to go through different stages. They deal with the treatment as they can. I encourage patients not to put their lives on hold. Often they say should I leave my job, should I rest a lot and we encourage them not to do that; maybe reduce the hours if they have really stressful jobs, but not to give it up completely because it leads to obsession about infertility and it makes it worse.'

This agonising time of fourteen days of suspended animation is common to all those wanting a baby, by any means. However, in infertility treatment, everyone has their recollections on getting through those days. And no one has an easy solution, as discussed in an earlier chapter. Most people simply wish they could go to sleep for fourteen days and wake up knowing whether they were pregnant or not.

Relationship with the Fertility Clinic

As in all human relationships, there are some people we relate to better than others. Clinic staff have to fulfil several roles. They must be the strict clinician, following the disciplines and ethics of the clinic scrupulously. However, they are also dealing with people in a life-crisis situation, so often they become the buffer between the patients and their doctors; the patient and their hopes and fears; and the official confidant if the couples haven't discussed their treatment with friends or relatives. Treading the line between clinical efficiency and general moral support is tough.

'It is difficult with DI because quite often couples are doing it in secrecy, so the normal support systems they have are not available to them,' said Eva Durna. 'If I know this is the case, I encourage them to ring the clinic if they have problems or feel

depressed. The most important thing is to get support. It doesn't matter where.'
Patients tell:

I think I gave over to them, I didn't really know what my body was doing, I trusted them — they had the machinery, I'm not medically trained.

The first clinic I went to I didn't feel they really knew — I mean they only tested me once a week then made a prediction about the day of ovulation. And it wasn't until I changed clinic and read the procedures at the new one that I realised they couldn't possibly have known. And they only did one insemination, not two, and after that no more blood tests to check on hormone levels or anything. They could never explain it, they'd just say not to worry about it. Not that I ever got down to asking exactly how, but I did try a few times to say how do you know. Apart from that, I just let them go ahead, they were the experts, I think that is how I've always been with medical professionals.

When I changed to the new clinic I felt they were particularly good to me, particularly efficient, because they wanted to do it quickly as I had already had thirteen attempts. I think they were quite competitive with the other clinic and couldn't wait to ring their colleagues at the other clinic and say they'd got me pregnant.

The good clinics give you a lot of information, which is great, but they should realise there is an awful lot to take in and remember. How can clinics expect you to remember all the things that are required of you without writing it all down.

Clinics vary depending on your interaction with the staff and the approach:

The first clinic I went to was OK and I conceived my first child. But the second one was a lot nicer and friendlier. I don't know that I can quite pinpoint the difference. In the waiting room at the first one, no one would even look at each other. It was not exactly cold, but certainly not warm either.

The clinic staff was always sympathetic, they are really in the firing line, not the doctor who you rarely see after your diagnosis is made and the treatment organised.

They were great when period time came. One even rang me back after I'd reported my period had started, to see how I was handling it, whether I felt OK or too depressed. I really appreciated that as I tried to keep a brave face for the rest of the world.

I refused to go back to my clinic while one sister was there. She once shouted at me in front of the whole waiting room. I was a couple of days overdue with my cycle, so I went to the suburban doctor to have a pregnancy test (you could do that then). The test had come back borderline, then five days after, my period arrived.

She just berated me saying don't you know we consider this as a pregnancy, a borderline pregnancy. We count that as a pregnancy. I told her no one had told me that and came away thinking this is just a numbers game for you — I'm a statistic on the board. Warren had to persuade me to go back, I nearly stopped at one child. I just wished she'd closed the door and given us all a bit of privacy. After that, if she came to call for the next patient, I'd give someone else my place and wait till the nice sister came (they alternated). I'd be a different consumer today.

—⁓—

Even though it was only a couple of months ago for me, still I found, even though I wasn't probably as vulnerable as the first time, I still wasn't as assertive as I'd planned to be.

Do patients share their hopes and fears in the waiting room? Leonie said, 'In the waiting room, I got chattier and chattier with each pregnancy. I got to know many women, but you could certainly get the vibes from those women who didn't want to talk.' Michelle added, 'If there were people there who'd instigate talk, I'd talk, but I certainly wasn't one to instigate it.'

If women won't confide in each other as they wait, do they confide their inner fears to the clinic staff? Eva Durna responded:

What everyone must realise is that women are not too open about revealing their problems to us because they're frightened we will say well, she's not coping well, she's never going to get pregnant, she's too stressed, she shouldn't be on the program and things like that. So they don't often talk about their anxieties and stresses to us. They don't want to be thought of as being weak, neurotic, can't cope, all those things. It's not good, not bad, if people can cope on their own. It's better than coming in crying all the time, so that's a different perspective.

The Pregnancy

'Once we get you pregnant, you go back to your regular obstetrician for the delivery.' These words from the fertility specialist come as a bit of a shock. Inwardly we rebel, thinking, but this isn't a normal pregnancy, it has been so hard to achieve. I still need special care. As the pregnancy progresses, however, you realise it is just part of the adjustment to life after infertility. Every child is special, but every conception wasn't this hard! This is common to all forms of assisted conception and many patients feel this sense of *abandonment* after their extremely close contact with the fertility clinic, its staff and their fertility specialist.

A Melbourne woman relates her experience:

After three unsuccessful cycles, the day came for me to change over to a proven donor. By this time I had become quite friendly with the clinic sister and she asked me if I'd like to go up to the storage area to collect the sperm straws. She carefully selected my allocated code and put some of it under a microscope to check whether it had thawed undamaged. She pronounced it not motile enough and rejected it. She selected another straw and let me look at a droplet of liquid with the wriggling sperm under the microscope. I had already viewed my mucus under the microscope. I was actually filled with awe that if this was the month for me to conceive, I had viewed some of the components which would make up our child. She told me not to waste this cycle, the sperm was really special. I found it amazing to be chatting about something normally so intimate.

That month I felt different. My temperature remained high at the end of the cycle and as I'd been pregnant once before, the symptoms were unmistakable, even before I had the test. It didn't stop the anxiety on the day of the test though. I thought I would burst if I didn't have it confirmed and went in a day early for the blood to be taken. I did get into trouble from the clinic sister for being so pushy, but I couldn't last another day. But the actual test result coming through was a bit

BABY SHOPPING

'I didn't frequent the baby shops till I was about three months pregnant, I was really concerned about buying stuff,' said Michelle.

~

'We had a great trunk of stuff Leonie had bought before we even found we had problems. She used to work in a department store. We even had four packets of nappies,' said Warren.

~

'I didn't dare even buy a crib for our baby till she was almost due. If she'd come very early it would have been a problem. But when I made a conscious decision to have a successful pregnancy a year before, I had bought an exquisite embroidered baby dress. So that would have been her only garment and she would have had to sleep in the washing basket.'

~

'We didn't do anything for our first baby for ages. I had bleeding in the first twelve weeks so I was scared it wasn't going to hold.'

~

'When we began infertility treatment, we tried three attempts at AIH. I was so optimistic that this was all we'd need that I went shopping for baby clothes. I had started this years earlier, but only when I saw something that was too adorable to miss out on. I have three large cardboard boxes of things hidden around the house. I am sure my husband doesn't know of their existence. After a number of failed ICSI attempts, I am now not so optimistic. I haven't bought any baby clothes for about a year now. Perhaps one day a charity group will inherit a number of cardboard boxes of yellowed baby clothes.'

THE BIRTH

'When I reached the end of the pregnancy the doctor began talking about induction. I said I'd had enough intervention at the start of the pregnancy and I wanted the end to be as natural as possible. He just looked at me as if to say *silly woman*. He then said he'd leave me with his registrar and walked out. The registrar was really great and said she understood why we wanted to have as natural a birth as possible. I couldn't in the end anyway, but I knew she only intervened when it was really necessary. She was quite happy to keep me in hospital as long as necessary. The other doctor couldn't understand why I wanted it to be natural,' said Caroline.

'I've heard it said that because you've been through the experience of infertility there is a higher incidence of post-natal depression,' she added, 'involving our very high expectations for parenthood. I know for years afterwards with Andrew, my first child, I'd tell him off then feel so guilty, thinking, I shouldn't be angry with this child, I wanted this child so badly.'

of an anticlimax, because I already knew. But it did cause some problems between my husband and I.

I was so scared it was going to be snatched away from me, I was too scared to make love. It was a tough time, which should have been joyful. He felt totally rejected and I thought he was a clumsy idiot not to understand my feeling of fragility. I was speechless when he said something like, 'Now you've got what you want, you don't want me.' Looking back, I should have given him more reassurance, but I expected him to be as happy and protective as I was.

'I don't think I even thought the first pregnancy was real — not even after the ultrasound. Not even when I was seven or eight months pregnant, I still didn't feel there was a baby inside me. I could feel the baby moving, but still I didn't feel it was real,' said Caroline. 'I was grateful for one useful piece of advice from the clinic I attended. They told me to request our baby's DI conception not be recorded on our obstetrician's notes. In this way, it prevents the general hospital staff knowing all our personal details when it comes to our child's birth and prevents gossip. Hospital staff are only human, and our need to use donor sperm was a painful choice, and a very private one,' said another woman.

Are there any specific problems with a pregnancy where the donor of the sperm is unknown? The following comments give some insight:

'I had one woman say to me that she thought she was carrying a monkey and another thought the baby didn't have a face — because of the DI conception. Then someone else who counsels with post-natal depression told me these were very common fears, even for women who conceive normally. I find that hard to believe,' commented Leonie.

'I had some very slight worries that the baby might be a different colour to us, though I had forgotten about this by the time of the birth,' said an English woman.

~

'I suppose the milestones were the same as with any pregnancy. The first scan showing the precious heartbeat, the amniocentesis, revealing everything was OK. I suppose the only real difference from a more usual pregnancy was that you couldn't sit and daydream about this small person being a fusion of you and your partner. Even though with an orthodox conception you cannot know about the baby in any real way, you do have all the basic genetic outlines. I didn't feel it was necessarily negative. In many ways it was exciting, as long as you trusted your doctor. Your baby comes to you as a total individual, without too many overloads of genetic expectations.'

The Last Straw

(or Donor Insemination in the Bad Old Days)

I'd been having DI treatment with a doctor in Harley Street, London, for about a year, I used to go every month when the temperature chart told me. This was fifteen years ago, so things have probably changed a bit now. So off I went for my treatment one Friday night and I was in this little cubicle surrounded by Arab magazines — because all the Arab ladies go to Harley Street gynaecologists — not a Woman and Home in sight, nothing worth reading. I had had my treatment, it was after work, so it was about 5.30 and you're always left there for about half an hour or so. After forty minutes, I thought, This is strange. It was very quiet outside. I left it another ten minutes (I'd been there about fifty minutes), then I thought this is definitely not right, so I scuttled off my little couch, went out and found everywhere dark.

'The receptionist had gone home, the nurse had gone home, the doctor had gone home, I was totally alone in this huge great building. And I thought right, I'm either locked in for the weekend or what, so I went outside, (properly dressed now, by the way) and there was nobody in sight. I trotted down the stairs and there was a porter who looked very surprised to see me. By this time, I'd gone beyond the disbelief. I was angry. Absolutely furious.

'My husband was waiting outside for me and he asked where I'd been. I said, "You won't believe this, but they've all gone home and locked me in." Then, when I had vented my rage, he said, "I thought you were meant to be calm for this treatment?" However, it was a free treatment. I phoned them up on the Monday morning, very cross with them, you can imagine, it wasn't quite the final straw, but almost.

Chapter 10
Issues for Donor-Conception Parents

'He's just like his dad ...'

~

'She's got her daddy's smile ...'

How many times are those observations made in the first weeks of your child's life? Parents of children born from donor sperm or eggs may think they will never get used to it, but oddly enough, after the first few months many find it becomes commonplace.

Whether friends know or don't know the means of conception, every new person seems to say it. As time passes, similarities of speech, expression and gesture do appear, so you can truly say your child is just like daddy — or mummy, if the child was conceived using a donor egg. The thing is, in donor families, this *is* the baby's father or mother. The donor is the donor, the parents are the parents. The distinction is clear.

After all, going through the pain of finding out you are infertile, making the decision to have a child using donated eggs or sperm, and going through all the tests and treatments to have this child are acts far more profound than the few seconds of orgasm taken to conceive most children.

Donor fathers discuss their feelings:

Early this year, my wife and I were sitting in the waiting room of our doctor's surgery waiting to see him for the 32-week check-up with our second child. As usual, he was running late and what was worse, I had been through all the National Geographic magazines in the place. Turning to my wife I noticed she had been studying the same folder for a while. It contained newsletters of the Donor Insemination (now Conception) Support Group. Little did I know what I was about to read was going to jump off the page and compel me to address issues I thought I had dealt with, resolved and banished to the recesses of my mind forever.

When I was sixteen years of age I found a lump on my left testicle. It turned out to be teratoma (a type of testicular cancer). The subsequent treatment left me free of cancer — and also my fertility. The doctor tried to make light of it, saying women hate taking the Pill. At the age of sixteen I had stumbled on the answer to the universe and gratuitous sex.

Five years into my marriage, we decided it was time for children. We had four attempts at IVF with my sperm, but finally they could not get enough sperm for

111

fertilisation. We chose DI. The day we decided on our donor I tried to imagine what he was like and what our child would turn out like. That idea was painful and one that I thought I could never resolve so it conveniently disappeared. The concept that replaced it was that of a faceless man with no emotions and lacking any desire to know what happened with his sperm, a totally benign entity. On one occasion I spoke to a doctor about my becoming the father of a donor child. He openly admitted he could not imagine what it was like to have a donor child as he was not even yet a father. He did, however, tell me about his brother who happened to be the father of a donor child. He said the question of whether it was his genetic child or not did not matter.

In the first two years of Nicholas's life, he was a total bundle of joy. Yes, I too did suffer from the not-my-child syndrome. At the moment I have on my desk all the child development and toddler taming books in the house and I have been through them all. It's 2 a.m. and still I have not found out what makes our two-year-old tick. I cannot understand how at this age he has completely analysed not one but two adults and he cannot even read yet. He is so good he presses buttons I didn't know my wife even had.

So it was when my wife was pregnant with our second child from the same donor that I abandoned the dog-eared waiting room magazine and flicked through the Donor Conception Support Group newsletters. It was the account of an experience of a donor that made me address my identity as father of DI children. As I read his story I realised he was not a donor, he was a man, a husband and yes, a father. Looking through into the future I hope that after my son has been through his adolescence, we might have a quiet moment when he will ask me what was it like to have a non-genetic son? My answer will be as a question, what has it been like to have a non-genetic father? I think by then we will both know the answer to each other's question. I think by then we'll have more in common than not.

Abridged from the *Donor Conception Support Group Newsletter*

At 19, I sustained a quadriplegic spinal cord injury and am now permanently in a wheelchair. Along with all the physical effect also came infertility. While I was not overjoyed about this news, it seemed less significant than some of the other bigger issues I had to consider. Right from the outset it was something all my family and friends knew about. I feel neither ashamed or inadequate because of it, and have always thought there was more to being a dad than biology and genetics — if only it were that simple. Don't get me wrong, nothing would please me more than being the biological dad of my kids, but it certainly wouldn't change the way I love and care about them. In fact, reproductive technology has come a long way since we had our kids, so now it may be possible for me to be a biological dad. The thing is, I don't feel the need to. In any event, I don't think I could perfect on what I already have.

Abridged from the *Donor Conception Support Group Newsletter*

A mother comments on the bonding experience between her husband and his non-genetic baby:

I was a little bit worried at the hospital, but then after being home about a week, suddenly my husband seemed to bond like cement with our baby. It was like that till one night he got very uptight, my family was staying with us, and those words I never thought I'd hear came out — 'Well, the child's yours, not mine, and you're kidding yourself if you think any differently.' I was shocked rigid. My chest felt like it would burst. The only thing I could do was go out and get in the car and drive somewhere alone. I cried, I raged inside. How could my intelligent, normally sensitive husband say something like that? He had been with me every step in the decision to have a baby by DI. It was the most committed thing we would ever do together. How could I ever forgive him? How could I go on? I felt so protective of my precious bundle — suddenly I thought of the baby as my sole responsibility. When I finally came home my husband had lifted the baby out of her cot and was holding her protectively in our bed. Did he mean it? I'll never know. My only mental retaliation was an inner sigh of relief and the thought, Well, at least I know she hasn't inherited your terrible temper. *But a degree of trust was shattered in me that night. A part of me will always be wary, no matter how wonderful their relationship is now our child is older. I really do know he loves her like he has never loved anyone in his life.*

Another woman, Mary, gives her view of donor conception and the concept of fatherhood:

We know the donor is the same height as my husband, the same blood group and hair colour as me and the same eye colour as both of us. He has achieved other pregnancies, something they were very concerned to tell us having achieved a previous pregnancy myself. We have decided our children will know their origins. They'll be told they have a very special daddy, and our niece will be told not all daddies are the same. I am happy to have only brief information about the donor. Our children will be just that—our children. I feel any additional information may cloud or complicate matters unnecessarily. As for the actual insemination, I don't have any definite feelings about the semen—it is almost irrelevant. What matters is that my partner is there to hold my hand, to give me my hormone injections if I need them, to take me to hospital when I need a late-night HCG injection and to hug me when I cry if they abandon a cycle. My husband says he's adopted a sperm.

Counselling

As assisted conception becomes more openly discussed in our society, counsellors will perhaps be assigned their correct role—as caring professionals who are there to help to work out a coping strategy for the couple. Up till now, they have more often been regarded as yet another obstacle to get through to assess whether couples are suitable to undertake procedures like DI.

The fear of showing weakness or wavering during any kind of fertility treatment is very real. The counsellor attached to a fertility clinic may be perceived by patients as someone who will report their *non-coping* to the medical staff. On top of this is the very real fear that they may be removed from the program, no matter how confidential the actual content of their consultations may be. And the dream of a baby would disappear. This perception must change.

'People shouldn't look at it as being a way to work out if they are going to be suitable parents, they should look at it as information and working out a coping strategy,' said Eva Durna, Senior Clinic Sister at the Royal Hospital for Women in Randwick, NSW, Australia. Couples explore their thoughts and experiences of counselling:

'I wish we had been told to go to counselling as a normal prerequisite. We felt they mentioned that counselling was available, but we sort of thought it was for people who couldn't cope and we were coping, we thought we were. I really wish we had been told it was part of the procedure. I wish they had considered talking about longer term things and what would happen after conception. We weren't inclined to talk about that, we wanted a baby at any cost, we would do anything to have a baby. I look back now and realise that was not a healthy attitude to have. I think in that position they have an obligation to you as a patient to hold the reins in, in a sense, to make sure you are counselled properly. In hindsight, I think the thirteen attempts we had before I conceived were really good for us. By the end of it we really knew we were doing the right thing. If we'd had success right at the very beginning, I don't know where we'd be today, I really don't,' said Michelle.

'It comes down to that informed consent business that is so talked about these days as far as the medical profession goes. I think most people, especially with DI, are not giving informed consent. You are not told all the emotional implications. More thorough counselling could assist in this,' added Leonie.

'Also, it's not just any counselling, but the right counselling. Like in any situation of crisis, the most helpful counsellor is one with similar attitudes to life generally as you. The counsellor attached to my clinic may have been very bright academically, but she was not very mature in real-life situations. I ended up having a fierce dispute with her over a moral issue. I thought she was incredibly naive and unworldly. She ended up adding immensely to my stress levels, not the other way round. I nearly had to change clinics because of her. So obviously I had no thought of confiding in her after that,' said another patient.

'At the obligatory counselling session before we went on the program, I regarded it as another test we had to pass to see that we were psychologically OK to be

parents of this child of the future. So it was a time of added stress, not stress relieving. I though if either of us mentioned anything bothering us about the whole procedure, or wanting to explore an issue, they would decide we were unsuitable, so we had to put on our perfect couple approach. I wanted a child so much, it never occurred to me to ask questions at that session about any implications of a donor child either on our relationship or on the child in the future. I think it is a hangover from the way prospective adopting couples are screened and the publicity which has surrounded that. You just don't think initially they are there to help you, you think they are there to judge and analyse your relationship.'

Family Secrets

To tell or not to tell? That is the question. The answer: it depends on the couple, their religion and beliefs, family factors, the child's personality. The only thing about the issue that everyone agrees on is that if a child is told, it must be done as part of a loving, intimate discussion with both parents — never revealed as an act of rage in a family quarrel. The doctors see this issue as one which must be determined by the parents and hesitate to give any set opinions. As the following patients tell:

'The doctor never commented on the fact that we were planning on telling our child of its origins. He said there is no need for anyone else to know.'

'No one asked us if we were planning to tell or not.'

Dr Stephen Steigrad, Director of the Department of Reproductive Medicine at the Royal Hospital for Women, Randwick, NSW, commented:

Less than 10 per cent of patients choose to tell their DI child of its origins and there is a lot of rubbish being spouted about this issue. There is a major difference (between DI and adoption). Half the genetic material will have come from the mother, so you know the background of that. Nowadays, being a bit more enlightened, we keep non-identifying information about the donor and he has been screened so there is going to be nothing significantly wrong in that background. So what are we trying to prove? Data from America shows that they looked at blood groups of mothers and babies and they found that in at least one group of hospitals about 10 per cent of the babies' blood groups could in no way have come from the fathers. So that is happening out in the community anyway. The big problem is who the couple have told. If you tell people you are going to undertake DI and the woman conceives, everyone will assume it's because of that, which is not unreasonable. Then you have a situation where other people know and the child doesn't. That's very dangerous (for the child). We had one couple and they'd told the whole street, then they proceeded to tell us they were not going to tell the child. We thought that was a bit strange. But of course they could move, we are a very mobile society. It is entirely up to the couple. Statistics tell us the longer people wait the less likely they are to tell. The easiest way is to say, 'Daddy's sperm was too weak so we had to use other sperm.' Quite often kids will say, 'You mean I'm not adopted?' Most kids go through a stage of believing they are adopted.

Warren's story:

After we found out I was infertile for a while we were still tossing up whether we'd have our kids by DI. Adoption was the only option and there was a ten-year waiting list — it's probably more now. For me that was not an option, the only option was DI. It took a little bit longer for Leonie to come round to that way of thinking. Before we actually decided to go down that road, Leonie decided she needed the opinion of someone else and so she talked to her best friend about it. At that stage when Leonie told me she'd spoken to someone else about it I was really angry with her — my main reason for that anger was that I've basically always thought that if you tell anyone else that the kids were conceived by DI, you must tell the child. Once anyone else knows about it there is no way it is a secret any more so that's basically the way I felt about it, so that's why I was angry with Leonie. Not so much that she'd spoken to her friend about my being infertile, it was that I felt we no longer had a choice in the matter now, we had to tell our children when they came. That was one little thing that happened to us along the way. I suppose I also think that people have the right to know about their origins, and if they found out later on it could have devastating consequences.

And others add:

'We certainly discussed it during my pregnancy and my husband said let's wait and see what kind of child we have. A lot would depend on the child's personality.'

'I suppose most of us pussyfoot on the issue because we are afraid of our partner's security and we are anticipating their very real fears of possible rejection once the child finds out.'

'I spoke with someone the other day who is planning not to tell her children. When I asked why, she said she thought it was to protect her husband. I said but if he's accepted his infertility and accepted his DI children, what does he need protection from? The woman said "That's a good question, I don't have the answer to that."'

'Are we supposed to be protecting this fragile ego? It's true, I wonder if that fragile male ego is a woman's invention anyway?' asked Caroline. 'I think telling them *was instinctive to us, we didn't want our child going through life without knowing about his background because it's his origins.'*

～

'One warning. It could be thought that, because there is doubt as to how a child may feel about being the result if AID (now called DI), it is better that these children should know nothing of their conception. I am sure secrecy is wrong. Family secrets have a habit of coming out, often at moments of family quarrel or crisis. Revelations of this sort would be devastating for most children and it must be preferable for them to understand how they were conceived as soon as they are able to comprehend the problem.'

Lord Winston, a leading fertility specialist in England, in his book *Infertility: A Sympathetic Approach*, Optima, 1994

～

'Say nothing. Let your silence be a gift to your husband. What is to be gained? You have a totally secure, happy child, why create doubts and uncertainties. Life is hard enough as it is, without that. Make sure you have absolutely nothing written down and ask that all the records be destroyed at the hospital. Anything written down is certain to be unearthed by curious little people,' said a psychiatrist with a European background.

～

'I just have this horror of how people with DI children go through normal family conversations, like who looks like who, and who gets what from which parent. There must be some awful silences when the child says, "Did I get that from Dad?" How can they get through those sorts of questions, they might lie. I'm sure a child can pick up on any hesitations and the fact that this is talked about differently to the way cousins and friends talk about things,' said Leonie.

Warren added, 'We decided to tell our daughter when she was about halfway through her first year of school, when Leonie was going back on the program to try and have our third child. Before we told her we were very nervous about it, we rehearsed for a couple of weeks what we were going to say. We put it off a couple of times. The night we decided to tell her we tried to make it the least stressful for her as possible. We got our other little bloke into bed early and we sat her on the couch between us.

'We basically told her how babies were conceived normally. How much of that she took in at five I'm not sure, she took in a bit. And we then talked about some friends of ours who have an adopted son and we said imagine how sad they must have felt when they found out that they couldn't have any babies. And how happy they must have felt when they brought their dear little boy home.

'We told her there are other ways of having babies, that she was born using one of these other special ways of having children. We told her we went to the doctor and found out I didn't have healthy sperm, my sperm couldn't make babies happen. And that we had to go to the hospital where we could get some healthy

sperm from a man who wanted to help people like us to make mummy pregnant. She took this in and thought about it for a while and then said I should go to a doctor so I could have healthy sperm. We told her we'd done that and that wasn't an option for us. The only way we could have babies was for another man to give us his sperm. Then she thought about it for a little while and said, "We should buy that man a present."'

〜

'I have a slightly different problem. I have twins from donor sperm and we do plan to tell them. But as one is a girl and one a boy, they are at different stages of maturity. At seven, the girl is mature enough to understand what we are telling her. Our son is not. So we have to wait till he catches up, to tell them together,' said a woman in rural Australia.

'Maybe the issue is not should we tell or not, but how do we tell, and how painful is this going to be for him and whether it's the right time. It depends on the sensitivity of the child,' said Eva Durna. 'As I can see it now, there are three groups of parents. The first group, they tell their children as soon as possible and they don't make a big deal about it. And the children, when they ask, they discuss it. Then there is the big percentage who don't tell their children at all, and that is over 90 per cent of people. And then there is a more radical group of people who want to tell not only their children, but the whole world.

'It also depends on the parents knowing their child. Every parent must have a moment when it flashes through their brain this is the way to tell this child. And if they don't have that moment of revelation, then there are always the books which have been written explaining their conception to children. The clinics and support groups can tell you about those, and they are written for very young children,' added Eva.

Patients comment:

'It will be interesting when our child is old enough to tell others, what their reaction will be. I feel very strongly that it is her history and her choice who to share this history with.'

〜

'I thought it was really funny when I read about the rights of DI children in England and that they have all the rights of a natural child, except they can't inherit a title. That seemed so very English.'

〜

'We don't have any substantial case histories about how donor offspring feel,' said the head of the Donor Conception Support Group. 'Of the three young adults who contacted us, all were glad they had been told. But the one whose father was a manic depressive had real problems. She was told when she was eight, but every time she wanted to discuss it with her parents her mother told her keep quiet unless she wanted to make her father sick. The father's attitude was, 'We've told

you now, that's the end of it.' What they didn't realise was that it was really only the start.'

―❦―

'One time when I was nursing my eldest daughter she said to me, "Mummy, who do I look like?" "You look like yourself," I told her. Then I looked down at her and said, "The donor must have been a very good-looking man, because you are a beautiful child,"' said Leonie.

The Professional Debate on Secrecy

Professor Ken Daniels, of the Department of Social Work at the University of Canterbury, New Zealand, has done some of the most extensive research and reporting into aspects of secrecy with donor children. In the August 1993 issue of *Politics of Life Sciences* (Beech Tree Publishing, Surrey, England), he co-wrote an article called 'Secrecy and openness in donor insemination', with colleague Karyn Taylor.

Within this edition of *Politics of Life Sciences*, other social scientists were invited to comment on his findings. The following selected extracts from these papers show the diversity of opinion worldwide, and the emotional minefield for parents trying to determine what is right or wrong for them and their children. Professor Daniels wrote:

The word secrecy has emotional and value connotations, the implication being that something shameful is being hidden from view. Perhaps the continuing desire for secrecy concerning donor insemination is not hard to understand when one considers that only 49 years ago an inquiry in the United Kingdom, headed by Archbishop Fisher, recommended that the practice should be considered a criminal offence.
Report of a Commission Appointed by His Grace The Archbishop of Canterbury, 1948

Daniels concluded:

Traditionally, the use of DI as a means of creating families has been shrouded in secrecy. Although there are increasing calls for more openness in the area, secrecy is still the guiding principle for many of those involved in DI today. The most common reason for attempting to maintain this secrecy is to protect the individuals involved. Secrecy is considered necessary: (1) to protect the child from stigmatisation and emotional trauma, (2) to protect the couple, especially the infertile husband, from stigmatisation and embarrassment, (3) to protect the donor's anonymity, thus ensuring there will always be an adequate supply of semen, and (4) to protect the medical professionals. It is important that questions are asked about just how necessary this protection is, and whether, in fact, it is more detrimental than beneficial to the parties involved. Research in the field of adoption, and early DI studies, have suggested that an open approach would be more advantageous to those involved in Donor Insemination. It has been repeatedly shown in numerous studies that deception and secrecy have a detrimental effect on family relations, and on the psychological well-being of the child. It has also been shown that there are practical difficulties inherent in trying to maintain a secret over a long period of time. Finally, it has become obvious that DI offspring have the desire, and the right, to know the truth about their genetic backgrounds.

Several social scientists responded. Rona Achilles from the Department of Public Health, Toronto, Canada, commented:

Perhaps it is because — despite DI's technical separation of sexual intercourse and reproduction — a dominant social meaning attributed to this arrangement remains sexual. The donor masturbates to donate sperm. A woman is inseminated with his sperm. Imagine an egg donor. The image is clinical (complex surgical procedures) and passive (eggs are collected). In contrast, the sperm donor masturbates into a jar. The egg donor's risks are physical and the sperm donor's risks are social. Culturally, masculinity, virility and fertility seem inextricably linked, and at times, infertility and impotence are therefore confused.

Professor Jacques Lansac, University Hospital Bretonneau, Tours, France has an opposite view to that of Professor Daniels, perhaps reflecting cultural differences and attitudes:

The aim of the centres [licensed donor clinics in France] is the treatment of human infertility of heterosexual couples. Everyone involved undertakes to respect the rights of the children to be born with one mother and one father. Embryos cannot be conceived outside the family context. If the couple is separated (death or divorce), the medically assisted procreation procedure must be stopped. In our French experience, only 10 per cent indicate they will tell their child of his or her DI origin. The majority of parents believe it is not in the child's interest to know his or her biological origins. The main thing for a child to know is that he or she was desired and is loved by his or her parents.

In natural reproduction, the child does not know the secrets of its parents. Perhaps he or she was not desired; perhaps his mother wept when she learned she was pregnant and considered having an abortion. In France, 10 000 births a year are as the result of adultery (three times the number produced through DI), and yet nobody claims that this should be revealed to the children. In our Latin society, fatherhood is more an affective than a biological role. Under French law, the father of the child is the husband of the mother. We do not agree with Daniels and Taylor when they write that the child (future adult) has largely been ignored in DI. In our system we respect the rights of children to be born with one mother and one father. Perhaps truth is not the same in every society?

Annette Burfoot, Queen's University, Canada, continued:

Men don't hide women's infertility. Women's infertility is highly visible when they undergo in vitro fertilisation and related procedures because of the lengthy, complicated processes the technology involves with women's bodies. Like men, women are judged in their failure to reproduce, not as an individual and named family head (carrying the family name), but as a member in the widely expected feminine service (to carry, to birth, to nurture). The male act of reproduction is seen as symbolically relevant to human history, while the female act is physically necessary for that particular moment in time. The good mother does have its own particular role in history, but is rarely noted individually.

Bartha Maria Knoppers, University of Montreal, Canada, suggested a middle ground can be found between secrecy and openness:

This middle ground would not force an identity upon any of the parties, but it does provide an opportunity to slowly remove the shame, lies, and deceit surrounding infertility treatment within the context of gradual social change.... Secrecy in families is socially driven. In our wish for greater openness, we should not single out the infertile and their families as a motor for necessary social change, but should rather transform those social attitudes that would have us believe that the gene is the person.

This debate is set to continue as long as there are new fertility frontiers being crossed.

Identifying or Non-Identifying Information

In the past, only sketchy details, if any, were kept about DI proceedings — either donor information or birth statistics.

It is now recognised that clinics and hospitals must keep careful records of all donors and their offspring. The length of time these records are kept changes from country to country (and state to state in Australia, the USA and all countries where there is no federal law covering assisted reproduction). The laws regarding records are changing constantly as parents lobby on behalf of their DI children to have registers of identifying and non-identifying information about donors kept.

In two Australian states, Victoria and Western Australia, laws have now been passed that children can seek the identity of their donors at the age of eighteen if they wish to do so. Donors must agree to this before being accepted on a program. This law also exists in Sweden. In most other countries, parents are given a brief outline of the donor's physical appearance and interests, but have no access to identifying information.

Until recently, there was very little emphasis on keeping these records — the only need foreseen was in case of a genetic inherited illness. But as with adoption, society has now become more open about all things, including the rights of children to know as much as possible about their personal histories. And some families have a very real fear of inadvertent incest among donor children.

We have nothing about our eldest child, not even non-identifying information. It was fifteen years ago and during the AIDS scare in the late 1980s and all records were destroyed. It is difficult for her when she has to do a family history at school. Then she can only do her social history. She does sometimes wonder where her birthmark comes from.

All I really wanted was a thumbnail sketch of the donor, his profession, interests and activities. If I had wanted a known donor, I think I would have been sophisticated enough to ask a friend I admired and liked to help us out.

Most clinics do now give a certain amount of non-identifying information and records are kept in case something happens in the future.

Dr John McBain, Clinical Director of Melbourne IVF, director of the international group for the study of female fertility Geneva and immediate past president of the Australian Fertility Society, had these things to say when interviewed on Australian television:

I feel DI will end up with a two-tier system. One tier will be a group of donors who are happy to be placed on a register for possible contact by the child when it is eighteen. This semen will be used with parents who plan to tell their child of its conception. The other group will be of donors who are happy to provide non-identifying information, but not to be identified. These will be used for parents planning not to tell, but who would nevertheless like some data about the donor. I feel people must stop using the comparison between DI children and adopted children. I feel very strongly about this. One of the major psychological difficulties for adopted children is the knowledge that they were rejected by their birth parents. Donor insemination children are entirely the opposite — they were very much wanted by both their parents, who went to great trouble to have them. That is a fundamental difference. Can a child really grow up insecure — knowing his entry into the world was such a longed-for event.

Dr McBain concluded:

I vehemently disagree with that (the comparison between donor births and adoption). With adoption you have a child that exists. There has been the gestation, the birth and the relinquishment of that child by the parents. The child can understandably wonder why they had to be relinquished, what were the dreadful circumstances. With DI the child doesn't exist, the child isn't there, the child comes into being by the use of anonymously — and generously — donated sperm. And I really think this is one of those instances where the best type of gift is anonymous. I see no allegory there whatsoever.

The Effects on the Parents

Four fertility units in New South Wales, Australia, participated in a recent survey with the objective to examine the psychological effects of donor insemination on couples. The questionnaire surveyed couples with DI children over a period of fifteen years. The results were as follows:

Forty-seven per cent of couples thought their marriage had improved, while 3 per cent thought their marriage had deteriorated as a result of having a child by donor insemination. Seventy-six per cent felt it had a positive personal effect and almost all couples had no regrets about having a child this way. More than 90 per cent of respondents felt very close to these children. In those who also had children not conceived by donor insemination (60 couples), men were significantly closer to their children by donor insemination than to their *other* children. There was a significant sex difference in perceptions of the child's resemblance: 61 per cent of women thought their child conceived by DI resembled their partner, while 89 per cent of men thought the child resembled their partner. Twenty-one per cent of couples were concerned about having to tell their child about donor insemination.

The conclusion was that donor insemination can have positive psychosocial effects on couples and close relationships exist between the parents and their children conceived by donor insemination. The concern about the physical appearance of children conceived by DI can be allayed with the finding that the majority of couples see a resemblance between the child and their partner. (Eva M. Durna, Judy Bebe, Leo R. Leader, Stephen J. Steigrad and Don G. Garrett, *Medical Journal of Australia*, September 1995; 163: 248–251.)

Divorce

It can happen — and what then for the bonding between donor sperm child and its father? One such father tells:

I'm the father of a donor child, and as complicated as those situations are, ours has another dimension to it. Three years after the birth of our son, my wife and I separated. I'm sure we're not the first and certainly not the last to experience this trauma. This separation has in no way weakened my love and commitment to my son; in many ways it has strengthened it. I look back now and think how easy it would have been for me to walk away from the situation and simply pay the required maintenance. This scenario never entered my head.

I have a very special relationship with my son; a bonding that grows stronger each time we get together. Ideally I would like more access to him and with time hope this will come about.

One of my early feelings in discussing the situation with the counsellor at the clinic was that we had let them down after all the work they had put into our situation. I no longer carry this guilt with me because I know of the very special relationship that my son and I are building.

Abridged from the *Donor Conception Support Group Newsletter*

Egg and Embryo Donation

This is a treatment for female infertility, where the woman has suffered premature ovarian failure, non-functioning ovaries, produces poor-quality eggs or carries an hereditary disease. As yet, the freezing of eggs is relatively unsuccessful, so originally in egg donation, the cycles of the donor and recipient had to be synchronised and the egg pick-up and fertilisation with partner or donor sperm completed and the embryos transferred into the recipient immediately they were ready.

In Australia, the same caution is now applied to the use of eggs and embryos as is used with donor sperm. As a result of the anxiety regarding the transmission of infectious diseases (especially hepatitis B and C, and HIV), it is required that the embryos resulting from donor eggs be stored for six months and the donor then re-checked to make sure there are no communicable diseases. Although the cycles don't have to be synchronised now, the recipient has to sit and twiddle her thumbs until six months have passed. If these precautions are not routinely carried out in the country where you are having treatment, it is worth asking your specialist for his or her advice and opinion.

Embryo freezing has a 60 per cent survival rate at thawing. Eggs are often donated by women who are undergoing IVF treatment themselves, and have surplus eggs. With

EGG DONATION

In the United States, egg 'donation' is becoming big business. As the 'donor' must undergo the same hormone stimulation and surgical removal of eggs as a woman on an IVF program, it is not as simple a matter as giving a sperm sample.

Advertisements for egg donors and fertility clinics are often placed in high-quality magazine such as the *New Yorker*, which is where I first saw them and felt vaguely puzzled. However, apparently the reader profile is correct and the advertisements are successful. Elite college newspapers are also used, as they circulate to a pool of healthy young women who may be likely to be attracted by the fee of US$1400 to $2500, and higher nationwide.

The costs of hiring an 'egg broker' range from US$8000 to $10 000 to recruit, screen and retrive oocytes (eggs) from a donor. With the additional costs of each IVF cycle being between US$5500 and $20 000, it is easy to see why the clinic advertisements are placed in magazines with upwardly mobile readers.

the refinement of embryo freezing techniques, couples undergoing IVF treatment may have surplus embryos after they have completed their families or stopped treatment. They can then donate these embryos to couples who cannot conceive their own.

Physically, this is not such a difficult technique: the recipient simply goes into hospital and has an embryo transplant at the time indicated in her cycle. She may have had drug stimulation to increase her hormone levels and increase the possibility of implantation. Emotionally, however, for both donor and recipient there are many factors to consider, and counselling is required to look at these issues before undertaking these procedures.

A donor shares her feelings:

I have just learned that my frozen transfer has failed. I feel very emotional about it, even though I have older twins from IVF with donor sperm. For five years I had known I had babies in waiting — frozen embryos waiting for me when I was ready. Now I am getting older, I decided it was time to have them transferred but they didn't implant. My added dilemma is that I donated the remaining embryos to a waiting couple. I just wish I knew if theirs had implanted or not — I think I wouldn't feel such a failure if I knew all the pain I am feeling for my failed transfer was turned into joy for a childless couple. But because of anonymity, no one will tell me. So I feel a double sadness.

These techniques are still too new to provide data on how these donated egg or embryo families are developing. In contrast, donor insemination has been around for many years, so it is possible to follow up on families and their children to assess their family structures and development.

THE DOUBLE DONOR
(OR DONOR EMBRYO) EXPERIENCE

Having a *double donor* baby leads couples into emotionally uncharted waters. There are no offspring from this technique who are old enough to comment on the effects of being told (or not told) about their conceptions, and few families have yet had the experience of bringing up a child who was born to them, but is the product of donor sperm and donor egg. Again, although adoption would seem to offer guide-lines, it does not, as children created through double donation are very much wanted and brought into being with great yearning, not surrendered at birth.

Alison and Peter, who live in England, answered my questions when Alison was in her sixth month of pregnancy, and agreed to do a follow-up after the birth of their child. Extracts from both are included because it is interesting to see changes in attitude once their baby was born. They differ from couples who have been given an existing embryo by donation. The sperm was chosen to match the husband, the egg that became available matched the wife. The embryo was created for them specifically.

'Because I was 45, we were given only one chance with IVF and were told that our chances would rise if we used a donor egg.

'This is a second marriage for both of us, and tests had revealed that I had blocked tubes, probably as a result of PID [pelvic inflammatory disease] from an intra-uterine device, and my husband had no sperm. Because of my age, a donor egg was suggested, which increased the chance from about one in twenty to one in three, but even with IVF treatment, we didn't really expect anything to happen. The treatment was so new in our clinic we had to wait ten months until the egg donation scheme was set in place. The donor sperm was selected from their *bank* to match my husband. By coincidence, an egg donor who was a good match for me came along at the right time.

'Counselling was offered and I did attend one session, but I'm not sure it was very helpful, although the counsellor was positive and sympathetic. We gained more from talking to others in the same position or with recipients of donor sperm. We went through a bad patch when we had to withdraw for a few months when my husband got cold feet about the implications of a double donor baby.

'I haven't had the baby yet. Maybe I will think more about how I perform as a mother than a normal mother. We do intend to tell the child about its origins, my husband in particular is convinced this is the right approach. But as donor children can't legally obtain information about their biological parents we do worry that we may have an angry, frustrated adolescent on our hands later on.'

Six months later, their baby is now a delightful reality. They both confess to being besotted by him, and now they share their views, knowing how it would have helped them to have access to people who had actually experienced a double donor birth. Alison says all the comments she makes are overridden by the fact that they both absolutely adore James. Any real problems centre on the issue of whether to tell or not tell their baby of his origins and how to deal with family relationships. Alison continues:

'The main problem, as we see it, is not whether to tell James (because small children can accept most things without question), but the effect on him as a young adult knowing he is not legally entitled to know where his roots are or *who he is*. This bothers us more than anything and was the reason we pulled out of the process for several months to reconsider. In the end we decided we just had to risk it. Sometimes we feel access to information about donors like in some other countries would be preferable, but that would perhaps cause other problems. Even if the law were to be changed in the future, it is extremely unlikely to become retrospective — and would betray sperm donors who donated on the condition they remained anonymous.

'The only parallel is that of telling an adopted child of its background, but even that is not the same because he can try and trace his natural parents. Then if that initial contact is not maintained, we are told the adoptee feels more at peace having met them. I read the other day that there is now a condition called *genealogical bewilderment syndrome* because of our advanced reproductive technology. But I don't know how seriously to take this, it may just be a newspaper slogan.

'It also occurred to us that he might as a stroppy teenager use it as a stick to beat us with, but we comfort ourselves with the knowledge that if it isn't that it will be with something else.

'It would be useful to see all this from the perception of young adults thus conceived, but of course none of them are old enough to make a contribution to the debate. Perhaps, with the decreasing male fertility we read so much about, by the time our child is grown up there will be enough double donor children to form their own support network. I feel we personally ought to know more about the psychological effect of *rootlessness*. Perhaps we will start doing some more reading on the subject.

'Other parents have told us that boys mature later and aren't often ready to be told till about seven or eight. I wonder if that is the age they also start worrying about being different from their peers. What happens when they do basic biology at primary school and our child knows he was conceived differently. Do I brief the teacher accordingly?

'The issue of "Who does the baby look like?" inevitably comes up. I think people always see what they want to see and quite a few think he looks like me. Surprisingly Peter's family have made no comments, perhaps because they are disappointed he looks nothing like them. If there were not a passing resemblance to me, we would probably have said when people asked, "Oh he looks a bit like so-and-so." Peter came up with a great line when someone asked him. He responded with "Well he doesn't look much like you, does he?" His colouring and general build seem about right, but a very close friend did say emphatically (and darkly) that he doesn't resemble anyone he knows. Actually, the clinic sister, having explained that because of the scarcity of egg donors it isn't usually possible to provide a match (unless you wait), then told us that our egg donor was a much better match for me than is the norm — not only in build and colouring, but she hinted, facially, too. When we pressed her, she said the donor was a keep-fit fanatic, and that also gives us a certain bond. I would love to meet her, or course, but she doesn't even know her efforts met with success.

'In retrospect, we feel we would have liked to know more about the sperm donor. Provision is made on his form to give information on his aptitudes, hobbies and so on, but the donor picked for us only provided physical information. Perhaps other couples could press for a donor who gave more detail, if there was a choice. It is likely ours was a medical student, but the clinic would not confirm this. I am not being ungrateful, it is just a slight regret.

'Another issue that remains unresolved is how to tell Peter's family. My parents are dead and my only close family is my sister and her family, and she's a nurse and thought it was all very exciting. Peter has an elderly father and his two sister's families to consider, all of whom we see regularly. We initially felt his father would find the idea either incomprehensible or distasteful, or both, so we waited until the baby was born, thinking something concrete would be more acceptable than a pregnant idea and that he would be won over by a charming infant. However, when we next considered telling him we realised that he was by then so taken with his grandson that he could well be disappointed to find that he is not genetically related to him and this is something we hadn't foreseen. It seems he was thrilled that it was a boy because the name will at last be carried on. His other grandchildren, coming from his daughters, carry different names. To someone of his generation this is important and of course I understand that. Perhaps he would view him as a kind of imposter. So until we tell him, we can't tell Peter's sisters, or we could tell them and ask their opinion. Everyone has to deal with this in their own way, depending on what kind of family they have.

'Certainly a plus point of double donor-ism is that we both feel equal, as would genetic parents. We have heard of the fathers of DI children sometimes feeling alienated as they don't have an equal genetic relationship with their child. We talked to one double donor mother who said they had actually chosen for both sperm and egg to be donated, even though his sperm was fine, so they had an equal genetic role. The only other similar couple we have met have not told family members because of problems within the family. There are very few people about who talk about their double donor children, and they never appear in the press, so we have very few comparisons.

'Finally, I have to say that James seems unusually sociable with a beaming grin he bestows alike on family, friends, total strangers and inanimate objects. He joins in with strangers' jokes and is a magnet for ladies' attentions when out and about. A friend says his eyes will cause women to fall at his feet in later life and this did occur to me, but then I'm biased. People compliment him on his beautiful hands, too, so we put ours in our pockets because they are square and stubby. We have found out that there have been two double donor babies born since him and maybe we will be able to meet those families. They have been born with the aid of eggs from family friends, which is a little different. Apparently it is almost impossible to get anonymous egg donors and we have nothing but admiration for the altruism of the few women who undergo all that hassle and stress for someone they will never meet, not even knowing if it will work.'

Chapter 11
Relationships

'There is no inner recess of me left unexplored, unprobed, unmolested.
It occurs to me when I have sex, what used to be very beautiful and very
private is now degraded and very public. I bring my report to the
doctor like a child with a report card.
'Tell me did I pass. did I ovulate? Did I have sex at all the right times like
you instructed me? Of course it changes your relationship with your partner.'
**The New Our Bodies, Ourselves, The Boston Women's
Health Collective, Simon & Schuster, 1996**

Infertility Is a Medical Condition

Doctors and hospitals exist to help people with medical conditions. The average self-satisfied comments from the fertile don't exclude people with perhaps self-induced HIV-positive status from treatment. They don't include stopping people having abortions in the health system (the argument has a re-run, saying we must stop the world from being overpopulated). They don't deny people with smoking-related illnesses treatment. Or other knowingly self-induced ailments.

For some reason, however, they feel free to moralise about the so-called selfishness of couples who want to have a family, as though they are asking for something luxurious — when it is something regarded as a right to most human beings. And whatever problems we have in conceiving are generally not self-induced ones.

In 1993, a division of Harvard Medical School and the Department of Psychiatry, State University of New York, conducted a survey to compare the psychological impact of infertility with other major medical conditions. The following is a precis of their findings. All the subjects were female, and they completed a standardised, validated and widely used questionnaire before enrolling in a group behavioural treatment program. The totals were as follows: 149 patients with infertility, 136 with chronic pain, 22 undergoing cardiac rehabilitation, 93 with cancer, 77 with hypertension, and 11 with HIV-positive status.

The infertility patients had global symptom scores equivalent to the cancer, cardiac and hypertension patients. The anxiety and depression levels were lower than those of the chronic pain patients, but not those of the other groups. The results suggest that the psychological symptoms associated with infertility are similar to those associated with other major medical conditions. Therefore standard psychosocial interventions for serious medical illness should also be applied in infertility treatment. (From *The Psychological Impact of Infertility: A Comparison with Patients with Other Medical Conditions*, by A. D. Domar, P. C. Zuttermeister and R. Friedman.)

Anyone who has suffered from infertility will know all this from experience. However, gaining the understanding of others as we continue with our *normal* lives is hard. Too often they imply we are using public money to buy ourselves an expensive bauble, not a much-wanted baby, and often we are paying privately at that.

Perhaps as there is more exposure to and education about infertility, more families and friends will empathise with the sufferers. And fewer instant experts will feel free to moralise. For we do have to continue our lives, whether we are successful in having a family or not. Like any profound experience, however, the quest changes us and our relationships with others — our partners, our families, our friends. The fertility clinic does become, for a time, the centre of the universe. They are involved with our most intimate functions, so it is not surprising that this happens. It is also a complex business explaining the intricacies of treatment to anyone not an aficionado.

In addition, many couples prefer to keep their treatment a secret, or shared with only a very few friends. Some, like the following couple, found they had a shared problem when they attended an information evening organised by a support group:

Only a few very close friends and my husband's brother and wife know of our problem. Strangely enough, all the members of our bridal party have infertility problems: ourselves, our matron of honour (unexplained infertility and many GIFT and IVF attempts) and my husband's brother. About a year ago I attended an information evening and I was surprised to see my brother-in-law and his wife in the audience. I discovered they were attending the same fertility clinic as we were for GIFT procedures because of endometriosis-related problems, and they were patients of the clinician right across the corridor from our own. Since that night we have developed a much closer relationship with them now that we have a special shared problem. My doctor tells me he experienced a similar coincidence with another patient when she awoke from egg pick-up in the bed next door to her sister, who was also recovering from the same procedure. The two sisters hadn't told each other they were having treatment. I have not told my mother because I know the news that we are actually planning to have a family would send her into a frenzy of bootee knitting.

Others have taken the reverse tack:

Once we decided to try DI treatment, we told everyone. I think they got a bit bored with us telling them month after month. I think one or two people at work thought I was silly to carry on and on and on trying. Now our baby has arrived they've changed their tune. I actually took my mum along to inseminations on two occasions when my husband couldn't attend, but she tended to stand in the corner so she wouldn't get in the way. The second time she came with me was the time it actually worked. It was great, she held my hand and gave me good vibes, it only took a few minutes, and we just made a bit of fun about it really. And it worked.

Relationship with Our Partner

All the sensitive doctors try and give you your fertility diagnosis without apportioning blame. However, because we are human and because we are going through a crisis situation, there will be times when your relationship is under severe strain — both physically and emotionally. Then it is hard to be a saint.

Maybe in some ways it is easier if you both have a problem, but of course that isn't always the case. Problems also arise when one partner has a child or children from another relationship. Then perhaps their need for a baby isn't quite so intense as that of the childless partner, so the infertility experience is tipped slightly off balance.

Most couples agree that when they do actually make it through to the other side of treatment, with or without a baby, their relationships are immensely strong. And as the previous chapter shows, surveys show that couples with DI children have a far higher than average rate of staying married than the rest of the community.

It takes dedication, intimacy and friendship to get through it. At various times along the way, one part of the relationship will suffer, only to be compensated for later on. While listening to my interviewees on tape, I marvelled at how these very normal couples could sit down and discuss the quality of the wife's mucus, or the state of his sperm, the developing follicles, the microscopic embryo, or how hard it was to get turned on for the post-coital test. To get young males, particularly, to talk with such intimacy and knowledge about subjects like this I felt was nothing short of a miracle.

Sexuality

While some doctors try to keep the subject firmly under control, concentrating on the scientific facts of reproduction, there iş no way to avoid the fact that semen, mucus, penises and vaginas are usually part of our private sexual experience, not something for hearty, open discussion. Equally, when something is found to be wrong with one of these otherwise sexual elements, the reaction is often a blow to the person's sexuality and sexual self-image. Getting through the initial testing, diagnosis and then the treatments takes great care, love and patience.

We all react differently:

'I do find that the treatment has a disastrous effect on our sex life — I vaguely remember having one once. But with all the prodding, poking, scans and speculums, I just feel totally violated at times. We've worked out our own ways around this — penetrative sex isn't all it is made out to be and there are other ways to make love that don't remind you of scans and speculums!'

'I went off sex for a while when I found out my husband had no sperm, psychologically feeling there was no point.'

~⦿~

'Our sex life has both suffered and improved as a result of our experiences. For a long time I felt I must be doing IT wrong because I wasn't falling pregnant and therefore I became intimidated by what I perceived as my lack of performance. At other times, particularly those times when I knew I was definitely not likely to fall pregnant, sex was a lot better.'

~⦿~

'Ordinarily my husband was the initiator of sex. During my fertile time, I felt I had to seduce him. What happened was we'd end up fighting, not making love.' He commented: 'It's pretty hard to get excited when your wife expects a command performance.'

~⦿~

'Our sex life was difficult when we were doing temperatures and having to perform on demand. But once we gave that away we were OK. And once I was pregnant, our sex life was just wonderful, that was the best nine months of my life. My partner wanted me to be pregnant for the rest of my life.'

~⦿~

'Finding out his sperm count was no good has had a disastrous effect on my husband emotionally, even though we had two other children many years before, without needing IVF. We have had a nil sex life since. He never discusses it. Totally nil communication. My mother-in-law is almost as bad. She doesn't believe this child is fathered by her son as she can't accept that her son is defective in any way.'

Emotional rapport with partner

The quality of the relationship between couples is under intense pressure, so it can easily split either way. Most men seem to be born with a deep suspicion of doctors and medical matters generally, so to be involved in a complex treatment is not easy for them.

Many couples also report that, except within the confines of support groups, there is really no place for the men to let off steam. They suggest that many of the counsellors are women, so men don't automatically let out all their fears and feelings to them, and they certainly don't admit problems to their more fertile friends.

So the couple's relationship itself has to be self-nourishing, and that is not easy, given the strain of treatment.

Women will usually choose at least one friend or family member to confide in, so they have an outlet. Also, as they are the ones physically involved in the treatment, women have the nurturing from the doctors and clinic staff to help them. For male-factor infertility, often the support groups, where men will find others in the same circumstances, are the only place they can let down their guard.

Some patients reported that their male doctors set up a private club atmosphere with their husbands; others the reverse, that their husband was made to feel like a fairly useless appendage. In both cases, you have to strive for more communication with the doctor and tell him if either of you are feeling left out.

Many couples find they reach a new level of closeness with their partner as they go through this intense experience together. For others, it only adds sometimes impossible strains:

I feel essentially Marc and I are very lucky, we have had the chance to go through so much together, and are now closer than we thought possible. In the early days it wasn't always so. While we were waiting for test results and the English health system, the strain was enormous. So we decided to find an affordable clinic while we still had a marriage to bring a child into. Now, we are each other's best friend, one seldom seen without the other. Our lifestyle is the envy of many of our fertile friends and family.

~e~

Emotionally, I'd say we have a very strong marriage. Four months into our marriage when Bruce had cancer it brought us together; being on IVF has made us even closer. I certainly felt he was very supportive of me during the first cycle. I feel he reached a new level of supporting me, which I probably hadn't felt in the past. He was happy for me to cry when I had to cry after that first pregnancy failed to develop. He didn't actually cry, but he was very sad, he was involved. I asked him if he felt he was being supported too and he said he was, so that was good.

~e~

All the investigations over the past eight years have taken us both through every possible emotion, stress and benefit our relationship could possibly encounter. We both feel our relationship is very precious because of what it has endured and now it is almost as if we believe it has had enough to cope with and we should work at making our life together as happy and wonderful as possible to make up for the sadness it has faced. It's kind of like treating the relationship as if it were a child who has survived a life-threatening illness. You recognise that each day is a gift with no certainty of tomorrow, but all the promise of the best day you can have today.

~e~

I come from a different point of view, this is my first marriage, but my husband has three children from his previous marriage. We already have a conflict before we start. It's not fair, he's already got kids, yet he can't now give them to me (after a failed vasectomy reversal). Unfortunately, the more times you have IVF, the more resentment builds up.

Tonight, there's a baby-sitter at home for his three kids. It doesn't stop me loving my husband, but the resentment is there. In the school holidays, I have to take care of his kids, then I hear them on the phone to their mother saying, 'Love you Mum, miss you Mum' and here I am, trying to have my own. We have the fourteen-year-old living with us all the time, and I'm dealing with these teenage emotions, while trying to deal with my own during treatment cycles. I'm supposed to give 100 per cent of my time to us being a family, but I feel I've done my bit, I want my child. It is becoming a barrier.

Another (drastic) solution:

I have a family in the UK—two teenagers—and had a vasectomy after their birth. When my current wife and I had been together for some time, we found we were experiencing difficulties with the divided families, so we decided to move to Australia, making our own roots together here. It is the best decision we could have made. Also, my case is different to many, because I stored some sperm before having a vasectomy. I actually bought a portable sperm bank and brought it over to Australia. That was an interesting story. We now have one baby from GIFT using the frozen sperm.

His wife added: 'In the UK all we had was his past and his life, we didn't have a life of our own. Now we do have.'

Rapport with Family and Friends

I didn't realise how remote from everyone I became during my treatment until taking notes to start this book. When I asked close friends various questions, they had no idea about my going off for blood tests in the mornings and the daily telephone calls to see what was happening to the hormones. I somehow mentally locked myself away, with my partner and the clinic staff the only people I really talked to about it. As I didn't have a long series of treatments and didn't have to have invasive procedures, I didn't have to involve others.

One very close friend and colleague, who had been in the same position a year before, shared my hopes and fears. I came back one morning and she had drawn the most wonderful swimming sperm and left it on my desk with a good luck message. But she was probably the only one, thinking back. And only because she understood, having tried for many years to have her second child.

My family didn't expect blow-by-blow details because I was older and independent, but that is not always the case. Some families can become very hurt if their daughter or sister shuts herself off from them: 'We feel so hurt that she won't talk to us, she doesn't want to visit us at all. She talks to us on the phone, but that is all.' The daughter adds:

*My parents are so pleased my sister is successfully pregnant, I can't face them with my own sense of failure, so at the moment, because I don't want to say anything hurtful to my sister, I am just better avoiding them, till I can cope better. I can't explain to them the pain I feel when I have a failed IVF cycle. I wish I could. There is so much of the technical stuff they just wouldn't understand.'

Other couples do the reverse:

We have both been very up-front about our search for our family because we believe it was not something to be ashamed about and because it was an is such an important aspect of our lives that by talking about it openly others in the same boat who wish to maintain their privacy will know they are not alone. This attitude did not gain us more support, in fact, I think it had the opposite effect.

Friends and family thought that because we were so open about it that we were more emotionally mature about the situation than we were, and often didn't realise we were still very raw with our experiences and hurting.

We found everyone would ask us about children. New acquaintances would ask did we have any children and when we said not they would ask why not. I think it is because of the exposure of infertility by the media, infertility has almost become the public's right to know — and to decide its ethics on the street.

———

We didn't keep our IVF treatment a secret, but I didn't get much support from friends or family. As we already had two children, one of each sex, none of our friends could understand my powerful need for a third child. They were very critical of me inflicting this treatment on myself.

It was hard to avoid criticism and negative comment, but I tried to remain positive about my passion to have this last baby. My older children went through my unsuccessful attempts with me and treasure their new sister as I do. In fact, they were more supportive than my husband. I felt strongly in the years to come that if I hadn't tried as hard as I could to have this baby, I would never have forgiven myself and could not have lived with my decisions not to go on as far as I could. I am so glad I followed my instincts — I have a magical two-year-old now.

Family Relationships

For some reason, your family is often the place you don't go to for support during infertility treatment. They are just a bit too close. Perhaps it is to do with sibling fertility, or perhaps it has to do with your mother's own fertility. Or perhaps, unless they have been through it themselves, they just simply can't understand why it is such an issue for you. No one can, unless they have experienced it.

They are either too concerned and worried about your well-being or not concerned enough. It is not their fault, but the fault of the emotional turmoil in which you find yourself. Just my mother giving away all my childhood books and my doll's clothes to my sister's children, assuming I was never going to have children, sent me into a fit of outrage. How dare she decide about my fertility? My feelings were not rational. Because my sister had difficulties having her elder children, I certainly didn't have problems with or resentment of her fertility. Nor did Christmases or family events bother me — I adore my nephews and niece, and as they were all born before I wanted my own children, they carried no burdens of envy. I just enjoyed spoiling them when I could.

In an ideal world, we would all talk about our feelings of envy or regret, but we seldom do, or seldom acknowledge feeling them, as this woman confided:

> My widowed sister became unexpectedly pregnant at 45, after a brief renewal of an affair. I was ferocious with her as I persuaded her that it would be ridiculous to add a new baby, unwanted by its father, to her responsibilities as a mother of teenagers. I thought I was being sensible and practical in my arguments, but I was also stern and unbending. In light of my sister's soft, compliant nature, one which had always looked to me for strength and guidance, I feel a bit guilty now. I was in so much pain wanting my own baby, I was simply determined she wasn't going to have this accidentally conceived last baby. But I couldn't see that all the practical advice I was giving her came from one source — envy.

Relationship with God

This is a testing time for anyone with a belief in the god of their persuasion. As we long for a child, we see atrocities each day on the television news. Starving children, abandoned children, children mistreated. How could a god exist and allow precious children to be born into this environment, while ignoring the love and comfort we could offer a new life?

Not only that, but some religions frown on reproductive technology, while some actually forbid it. So for those couples, as they seek comfort in their quest for a child, the place they usually find comfort — the church — is denied to them. They are on their own with their consciences. Just as the laws of the land are struggling to keep pace with reproductive technology, the laws of the church, often decades behind in other matters, haven't even begun to debate the issues in a modern way.

One woman tells:

> I am a Christian, I do believe God has things under control, I do believe He is the giver of life. I know that if I can't have a child I will have to accept that is His will for me, but I also see no obvious reason why He wouldn't want me to have a child. I was also wondering about my parents' reaction to IVF and the reaction of my parents' friends. Whether they would think we were fiddling with nature, killing embryos and things like that.
>
> My husband and I have taken the attitude that God gave us modern science and the brains to work out treatments for infertility, just the same as He gave modern science the ability to take out an appendix, administer chemotherapy, do a hip replacement. The thought of not having a child I can't fathom at all. I would try every single thing I could think of, every way to get a child if I couldn't have one by IVF. I would find it hard to accept if that's what fate or God had handed out to me. But I suppose I would have to accept that.

DONOR INSEMINATION AND THE CHURCH

An ordained minister, father of two children by DI, which is against his church's teachings, searched for his own answers:

My church was opposed to DI and it suited me, as I didn't want a child at that point, fathered THAT way. We were going through the process of overseas adoption when we found out about the possibility of adopting an embryo, which I, and my church, considered favourably. But there was a long wait and only a slim chance of success. This got me thinking about DI again. Our specialist was very kind and patient and often our appointments were 10 per cent medical, 90 per cent ethical. With some prayer and struggle, we went ahead with the DI program. I had to work out the God-and-me issues myself. My denomination doesn't approve of any reproductive technology which deprives the child of its genetic heritage of its two parents who are to have social care and responsibility for it. Some ethicists liken it to a kind of adultery, with the introduction of a third party into the marriage covenant.

I was reading about Liberation Theology where the priests in Central America practised their theology through the eyes of the poor. So using their principles, I began reading the Bible through the eyes of the infertile. These were some of the points I made:

- In Genesis, God says to the men and women He had created, *'Be fruitful and multiply.'* So to want to have children is not a selfish urge, or keeping up with friends, but a basic primeval urge put there by God himself.
- What is the origin of infertility? Biblically, it is called sin. It brings deep sadness to those involved. But why is it that those who pontificate that it is God's will that couples should remain infertile, then have their children vaccinated against all manner of diseases. Surely these diseases have the same foundations in God's will. They go to a doctor if they become sick, but infertile people are not allowed to seek the same medical expertise to help their disease. DI is nothing like adultery. I was in the room with my wife when she was inseminated. We committed ourselves to it and went through it together. The Bible says in marriage, the two become one. Through marriage, I share in every aspect of our children's conception, gestation and birth and development. The church often says the infertile have a choice to serve in the community. In the gospel Matthew, Jesus speaks of only a few people being able to survive celibacy (read childlessness) for the sake of His kingdom. I don't believe He was talking about the one in seven couples that experience childlessness through infertility. I feel some church hierarchies have added to the suffering of infertile couples.

I cannot say I feel totally comfortable in making a choice that goes against the ethics of my own and most orthodox religions. I know my theological reasons may be shot down by the letter of the law, but by the spirit of the law my reasons are right.

I sometimes still struggle with my infertility. But it drifts into the background when I hear those beautiful words from my daughter — 'Me love daddy' — for they may have a donor father, but I, and no one else, am their daddy. Nobody, or their opinions, can take that away.

How To Answer the
Question 'Do You Have Any Children?'

Anyone who has experienced sub-fertility or infertility knows this question is a minefield. We all work out ways to deal with it. Depending on the sensitivity of the questioner, they accept your stock answer or they blunder on, ignorantly pressing on countless wounds, repeating the tired old cliches.

I said I had magazines, not babies. Others say:

We say we're still practising.

I used to find it easier to say I don't like children. It hurts as you say it, but you're going to get hurt anyway.

Because in the first few years of marriage we didn't want kids, some of our friends think we still don't want them. It is only in the last six months we've told people we are having our first IVF attempt. I found finally it was easier to let them know than having them say why aren't you having children. If they knew you were having problems, then they wouldn't ask.

We've heard some funny answers given to this question: 'We don't really believe in sex after marriage. We didn't realise it was compulsory. We're gay; what I mean is we're very happy as we are, thank you.'

Our line that worked best for us was 'It's not that easy for us.' People shut their mouths very quickly after that.

In my research for this book, the line I thought most effective was 'Sadly, no.' It seemed to cancel any of the ready cliches from the uninformed and positively to discourage further probing, except from close friends.

And of course, all people who have experienced infertility will confirm it is the one question they never ask anyone!

Chapter 12
Nature's Way —
Complementary Treatments

'We are on Chinese herbal medicine at the moment. Walking
through our house it smells like a deep, mossy valley.'

'I went on all sorts of diets and finally I said I'm sick
of this bloody diet, just give me grog and ice cream.'

'I've got into mind power and I really think it helps a lot.'

One of the most frustrating things about infertility is the knowledge that achieving your
dream — a child — is entirely beyond your control. On the one hand, the doctors and
fertility clinic are monitoring and controlling the scientific aspects of conception. On the
other, God or destiny appear to be controlling the less scientific parts. As the person in
the middle of it all, often your body and your emotional core seem unsynchronised, even
disassociated.

Many of us seek the help of natural therapy practitioners, who are trained to treat
the body and mind as a whole entity. By doing so, we gain back some control of our
bodies and our lives, and feel we are actually doing something to assist the doctors and
scientists — and ourselves. If we can make our whole being as pure and receptive as
possible to a pregnancy, perhaps our longed-for baby will eventuate.

I sought the help of my valued chiropractor and friend Leonie McMahon, who had
healed my damaged shoulder a few years earlier, and whose range of natural healing
skills, including acupuncture and homeopathy, had guided me through many a personal
and professional trauma. It was she who sent me to the doctor who was then practising
a controversial therapy of vitamin C intravenous drips to cleanse the body of toxins,
including lead. Leonie felt he may be able to help me detoxify, or at least identify any
toxins, so that I could maintain the next pregnancy I achieved, after my two miscarriages.

As discussed in my introduction, the doctor sought information surrounding my birth
and then suggested I think more seriously about the fact that I had been born in
traumatic circumstances and my mother and I had almost died. It was he who told me
about the influence our unconscious mind has on important issues in our life, and he
who suggested I try self-hypnosis to *un-learn* whatever negative residue I stored from my
difficult birth. I had been to a hypnotherapist in the past to learn relaxation techniques,
so I used a little of both, knowing it certainly couldn't do me any harm.

I was mystified by my miscarriages and as no one could give me any explanations except that they were glitches of nature, I wanted to try get my body and mind in top order if there was a next time.

I was encouraged by a fortune teller who told me in my early 20s that the souls of two sons had chosen me as their mother and would wait for me to decide it was time for them to come into the world. Any positive vibes helped. Another clairvoyant, just a month before my son's conception, told me the same thing; he also told me the precise number of previous pregnancies I'd had and explained I'd been a bad mother in a former life, so I was born with the desire for children, but I wasn't allowed to have them until I learned from loss to appreciate them. The next one, a son, I would be allowed to have, I could also have another son. After that I would not be allowed any more as I would go back to my bad habits. At least I was encouraged that he saw living children there.

What we'd all be too embarrassed to explain to doctors is that, given the fact that everything scientific is being done for us and it isn't working, we ask why. No one can help with that question. So depending on our personal beliefs and our particular level of desperation, we do seek alternative answers. From empowered crystals to crystal gazers, from renewed faith in God to plea-bargaining with all manner of gods, like me.

Natural therapies, with all their scientific and traditional roots, fall somewhere between the strictly scientific approach and the metaphysical. They vary in fashion at different times, but most natural therapists try to treat the whole person, not an isolated medical patch within that person. The treatments most commonly referred to by patients in my research for this book have been:

- chiropractic/osteopathic to balance and align the body correctly, ensuring proper blood and energy flow and stimulating the nerve supply to the organs;
- acupuncture to rebalance the energy to the hormone systems;
- homeopathic dilutions to prepare to raise the energy for the reproductive systems;
- herbal medicine and Chinese herbal medicine;
- hypnotherapy and/or psychotherapy;
- visualisation;
- massage and aromatherapy.

Of course, good nutrition is a prerequisite for anyone seeking a pregnancy. Doctors and natural therapists are in agreement there. Maintaining a healthy weight is also a prerequisite. Being overweight may make you produce too little progesterone; being too thin can mean you produce too little oestrogen. The correct balance of these is necessary for healthy menstrual cycles.

Timing of intercourse is also the most natural of therapies, and while the doctors may suggest you take your temperature to determine when ovulation occurs, indicated by a tiny dip then a rise in temperature, or use a home ovulation testing kit to gauge ovulation times, natural therapists will also start treatment by checking that intercourse is occurring at the right time. They may also suggest the methods above, but they will probably ask you to try to get to know your vaginal mucus patterns. The mucus at ovulation times should feel *stretchy* when you place some between two fingers and separate them. The texture should also be more slippery, rather like the sensation of raw egg white.

I had bought the book *The Billings Method* which pioneered the use of vaginal mucus to determine fertile periods, but I have to admit defeat — I could never really get the hang of working it out. Now, long after I need to know about ovulation, I am aware of the changes mid-cycle and also the increased sexual desire at that time. In those days of wanting a baby, however, I was so immobilised by need, I couldn't read any signs. My imagination was so overrun by signs, symptoms and portents, the natural rhythms of my body and sensuality were numb.

Some women are happy to let the fertility specialist do his work and do not need to do anything themselves to assist the process. However, many feel the need both for empowerment and to take charge of at least one aspect of their lives within this complex process. Sometimes we tell our doctors we are consulting a natural practitioner, sometimes we don't — perhaps for fear of being laughed at as the chasm between formal medicine and natural healing is still wide.

Most of the doctors I interviewed accepted happily that their patients may do extra things like massage, aromatherapy, acupuncture or hypnotherapy to aid relaxation. Usually, however, they preferred that the patient didn't actually take anything orally that may conflict with the treatment being given, or harm or interfere with a possible pregnancy.

There is an unanswerable, but universal question patients ask, which goes something like these words from a woman on Australia's Gold Coast:

Do you know what intrigues me? I've written down here don't eat ice cream, because you should keep your body warm, don't eat bananas, only have decaffeinated coffee, no cigarettes or alcohol. It still amazes me — we try and do all those things, often taking horrible herbs in conjunction with these restraints, yet still heroin addicts and starving people in Third World countries conceive, 16-year-old kids who eat junk food and get drunk are falling pregnant. How can that be?

Unfortunately no one has an answer, but we keep on trying. One patient said, 'I felt I'd donated my body to science', as the things the doctors were doing as part of her treatment felt so unconnected to her. This was not said as a criticism, but as a statement of fact. The complexities of assisted reproduction can make people feel that they are simply providing the raw material.

'Because conventional medicine hadn't helped and I hated the drugs associated with my one failed IVF attempt, I went to a homeopath, basically to help with my painful periods. I found it so beneficial, a homeopath looks at the whole person. My periods became less painful, I stopped work to lower my stress levels and within a month I was pregnant naturally with my son,' said a patient in London. 'Unexplained infertility like mine is, I believe, explainable. Doctors have one answer to a whole range of problems, but I believe with women there are lots of psychological and emotional issues that can't be solved by chemicals.'

In my case, I felt I had to try to work on several things in my own life, to try to help the doctors and myself the next time I was pregnant. I finally acknowledged my stressful job and work-associated travel may not be conducive to a pregnancy, so I started swimming in the mornings to relax, had massages when I could and cancelled any interstate meetings in the second half of a cycle, as I'd read air hostesses had a high rate of early pregnancy loss. I made sure I didn't take alcohol or even aspirin in the second half of a cycle, in case it harmed an embryo that may be developing (probably a bit extreme, but I was determined I wouldn't do anything that could be harmful to a new pregnancy). I even stopped drinking tea and coffee containing caffeine. I never did get used to decaffeinated tea.

Perhaps another thing we don't confide to the doctors or clinics is the level of our guilt and self-flagellation when we do conceive and lose a pregnancy. The endless 'if onlys' are tortuous, so even if what you are doing is scientifically unproven to help, if it makes you feel you have done all you can, it stops some of the self-torture.

Combined Natural Therapies

After my second miscarriage I took myself back to my chiropractor to ask her advice. Leonie McMahon is at the top of her profession and is trained in many natural disciplines — chiropractic, osteopathy, homeopathy and acupuncture. She is the author of two books on natural healing (*Why Am I So Tired?* and *Freedom from Pain and Distress*, Pan MacMillan, 1995). She works looking out onto her leafy garden in a peaceful suburb.

After the miscarriages, I was feeling fragile and empty. Leonie immediately prescribed homeopathy for shock. When I was ready to start again, I went back to see her.

First she explained the importance of pelvic alignment, as indicated by leg lengths. If one leg is shorter than the other and there is no physical abnormality, a chiropractor will suspect that pelvic alignment is uneven, she explained. It can also be indicated by a standing X-ray, but if someone is wanting to have a baby, X-rays are not a good idea, so leg length can be checked by lying flat on the treatment table.

The pelvis can go out of alignment as the result of a simple fall at any age, falling on the hip when you are younger or landing flat on your bottom. You can also easily suffer joint sprain and become unbalanced through normal activities such as sitting incorrectly, sleeping on a poor mattress or from accidents large or small. Emotional stress will aggravate your weakest area, creating physical tensions that affect the shape of our bodies (like curved spines, tilted heads, dropped shoulders and uneven hip-lines). Your tailor will tell you about your shape quicker than anyone. The importance of this pelvic alignment is that it affects the blood flow and the nerve supply from the back to the female organs. It will also make subsequent labour extremely painful and long.

Once the pelvic alignment is expertly corrected, Leonie tries to establish the menstrual history of her patients — at what age their periods started, how regular they are, whether they have a natural flow, are not too long or short, and not too heavy or heavily clotted. She prefers them to last about four days, with a light start, a flow and a lighter end. She said it was also important to establish whether patients had other symptoms like breast tingling, PMT or breast or abdomen swelling. In some cases, vitamin therapy is suggested to balance the hormones. In other cases, homeopathic treatment or acupuncture. As she explained:

In acupuncture, you must look for the balance of the spleen meridian. The earth pulses on the inside of the leg from the inner ankle control the hormone balance and the flow. You can stimulate these before a pregnancy begins, but cannot afterwards, for fear of starting the baby coming.

For people with recurrent miscarriages, she finds it is often because there is *rubbish* on the lining of the uterus. For my fibroids, she suggested fasting on juice from 4 p.m. one day till 4 p.m. the next day for a 24-hour period each week, until there was a shedding from the uterus, unrelated to my period.

So, in the total analysis, acupuncture is important to balance the hormones, chiropractic to keep the pelvis straight, and controlled, modified fasting to purify the uterine lining. Leonie goes on to say:

But the pelvis is so, so important. You are looking at the base chakra, within it all your attitudes about sexuality and who you are and your experiences through life.

I would add one further thing here. I now also look at the neuro-emotional field, and I go back through patients' lives to see if they had any unhappy experiences, be it from birth or childhood, or some sexual experience that may. have put them off, so I get them to talk about those things while I work on that area. Sore places in the body are often emotional blocks caught in the physical body.

I had a woman who came to me a little while ago who had been trying to have a baby for several years. She had a challenging job which was stressful, but which she loved. As I massaged her, I asked her to tell me what was the most important thing in her life. She said, 'I don't know.' I said: 'You don't know. I thought it was to have a baby.' She promptly burst into tears and walked around the block.

When she returned, she told me she was really frightened to get pregnant because she thought she would make an inadequate mother. I gently explained that all mothers have this fear, but that we learn as we go. Our children teach us, not the other way round. She was pregnant very quickly once that subconscious stress was removed.'

Do holistic practices work and, if so, how do they work?

Chiropractic

In the chiropractic discipline, body alignment is crucial. Because our bodies are highly flexible for ease of movement, they can also become unbalanced through normal activities like sitting incorrectly or sleeping, or from accidents large and small. Emotional stress can also create physical tensions that affect the shape of our bodies. The longer we remain out of alignment, the more our movement becomes increasingly restricted, and the resulting physical incapacity can also affect our emotional fluidity. Chiropractic is the most popular of the various methods of realignment.

The practitioners believe that the spinal column is the key to the nervous system, and they make expert adjustments, gently moving the vertebrae to restore nerve function and lymphatic flow between the brain, muscles and pelvis. They believe when proper nerve function is restored, the organs will function more completely. Hence Leonie McMahon's emphasis on pelvic alignment for correct nerve and blood flow to the female pelvic organs.

Homeopathy

Homeopathic treatments use remedies from natural substances diluted by a special method of serial dilution. The basis of this treatment is an ancient one dating from Hippocrates in 400 BC, which was called The Law of Similars, or *like cures like*. So by treating a fever with a fever-inducing natural substance, you cure the fever. In the early 1800s, a German physician demonstrated it was possible to cure without significant side-effects by using a very small amount of the appropriate substance. So he developed the technique of serial dilution combined with chemical agitation. Treatment with homeopathy is the least spectacular form of therapy. The tiny white balls impregnated with the specific distillate of the healing substance simply taste like minute sugar balls. Homeopathic remedies also come in drop form.

I was amazed to find while living in France that most of the local doctors there have certificates on the wall also stating they are doctors of homeopathy. This seems to be one country at least where ancient and modern medicine coexist harmoniously.

Acupuncture

Acupuncture has become more respectable with the general medical profession, especially since the opening up of China and the increased awareness of acupuncture uses and techniques even during major surgery. There was a minor wobble in the early years of HIV awareness, but practitioners began to use electric pulses instead of needles on the acupuncture points to avoid shared needles or to have patients provide their own needles, or to increase the sterilisation capacity for needles in their clinics. Now practitioners mainly use disposable needles. For at least 2000 years acupuncture has been central to traditional Chinese medicine. The classic philosophy of Taoism in China promotes maintaining balance in the body, and the belief that the body has the power to repair, regenerate or restore balance. Through acupuncture, it is believed the body can stimulate or awaken its natural healing powers. Yin and yang are the words most commonly associated with the practice. Yin is the *negative* (the earth, the moon, coolness, moisture, female things). Yang is the *positive* (sun, warmth, dryness, movement, things male). The terms are not aimed at being sexist, just the equivalent of positive (protons) and negative (electrons) in modern physics.

Unlike Western medicine, anatomy wasn't the basis for medical understanding in the Chinese. As ancestors are worshipped, dissection of bodies wasn't permitted, so research and treatments had to be based on other aspects — like the life *force*. They call this force the ch'i. They claim this ch'i circulates in the body along precise pathways, the acupuncture meridians. This life force must flow freely along these channels for all the organs to function effectively. If it is blocked or impaired, a person becomes susceptible to disease. Stimulating along these meridians controls the flow of ch'i, moving energy to deficient places, unblocking blockages. A traditional acupuncturist makes a diagnosis by examining the twelve wrist pulses, looking at the tongue and listening to breathing and voice patterns. The sterilised needles used are so fine they are practically painless and cause no bleeding.

Visualisation

Visualisation is a somewhat trendy term for synthesising our hopes and dreams into a tangible statement and projecting it into the future. What it really means is creating a positive image of what we want for the future and focusing powerfully on this, especially in difficult times. Because there is such a feeling of failure surrounding infertility and its treatment, any positive thoughts have to be good. The feeling of failure is made more profound by the knowledge that many other *less worthy* people we know seem to conceive effortlessly. Also, in an effort to avoid the monthly disappointment, patients often force themselves to be negative to minimise the despair when their period arrives.

Visualisation techniques date back to the earliest healing practices in Babylonia and Sumeria, and many ancient races have used these techniques, as well as indigenous peoples in more recent times. Placebos sometimes used in medicine today are a form of visualisation, as the patient imagines the medicine they are taking will cure them, therefore it does. Visualisation itself requires relaxing, feeling at one with your projected image of what is to happen, and focusing completely on that one thing, to the exclusion of everything else. Two successful recipients of IVF treatment describe their experiences as follows:

> *I kept trying to stay positive, to keep the negative thoughts away. I got into mind power and I really believe this worked for me. I used to do visualisation every morning and every night. I'd spend 15 minutes quietly sitting down totally concentrating on a baby being in my stomach. I'd think of it as a growing human being and imagine that I was actually pregnant at the time I was concentrating on it. Surely enough, I did get pregnant.*

~

> *I used that, too, but not as formally. But the same sort of idea and many people I've talked to did so as well — positive thinking and visualisation really helped. I*

made up a line for when I was driving around, something like the embryos were going to implant and IVF was going to be successful. I kept repeating it and repeating it all the time. It really worked.

For me, I used my vitamin doctor's suggestion of ridding myself of any negative residues from my birth and absence of younger siblings. It was like a mantra and went something like, *Hello, my subconscious, could you please contact our inner self and retrain it not to have fears and negative thoughts about pregnancy and childbirth.* Like the others, I found it an affirmation that one day I could have a successful pregnancy. Also, for me, buying nighties with a front-opening for breastfeeding to take to hospital was a real act of declaration of war against infertility. I did this just before I entered the formal fertility program, and this was also a kind of positive projection. I badly underestimated the size though, and they didn't actually make it into the obstetrics ward with me, but the sentiment was good at the time.

Herbal medicine

Within this section, two types of herbal medicine have to be discussed:

- the more traditional Western supplements, like those available in pharmacies, health food stores and from your natural health practitioner; and
- loose herbals such as those used in Chinese herbal medicine, which require a brewing of the prescribed herbs and drinking the liquid.

Each method has its proponents and detractors. The medical profession is generally cautious about the use of herbal preparations. Since the drug thalidomide was widely prescribed and found to produce severe birth defects, doctors have been anxious about pregnant or potentially pregnant women taking any kind of medication, natural or otherwise.

The vitamin folic acid is the exception to this. Meticulous medical trials have established that if women take folic acid — a B vitamin — before they conceive and for the first twelve weeks of the pregnancy, it can prevent diseases of early development like spina bifida, neural tube defects, deformed limbs and mongolism. Your doctor or health practitioner will suggest the required amount.

'Herbal medicine has been practised since time immemorial and is the basis for all pharmacopeia,' said Francesca Naish, a naturopath. 'Herbs are very powerful and gentle in their action, and can be used to treat both acute and chronic, short-term and long-term conditions. Because they have traditionally been dispensed by women practitioners, there is a wide range of herbs available for treating reproductive and fertility problems.' (From the ACCESS Fact Sheet *Natural Medicine and Fertility*.)

'Once a pregnancy is confirmed, some women crave specific foods, and it is fairly obvious to a natural practitioner which vitamins or minerals are needed. I was eating up to ten oranges a day at one stage in my own pregnancy, and it didn't take long to work out I needed more vitamin C. Similarly, when I craved bread, I knew the B vitamins were deficient,' said Leonie McMahon.

'When I prescribe herbs, I use prepared herbs in capsule form from a reputable company,' Leonie added. 'Although tablets are not as effective or direct (as liquid herbal preparations), they taste better and you know they are safe. They have gone through the *Therapeutic Goods Act*, and you know the exact dosage.'

Chinese herbal medicine is becoming increasingly popular, and one group of couples interviewed spoke very highly of the results. Within the specific benefits from the herbal therapy, they also spoke of their sense of well-being with the practitioners who treated them, who took time to know them and talk with them, whereas in a busy fertility clinic time is not always available. The clinic counsellor often sees so many people they have no clear memory of individuals or their cases, whereas the individual treatment from the natural therapists was almost as critical as the treatment itself.

A Queensland patient relates her experience:

'*Our house smells like you are walking through a deep, mossy valley it is so full of Chinese herbs,*' said one Queensland patient. '*The woman I go to is actually Chinese, she writes everything in Chinese. She told me she would take my problem to the professor next time she went to China. I'm seeing her more for well-being really, and to try and balance out all those IVF chemicals I'm taking. She can't really figure out why I'm not conceiving.*'

Her husband adds: '*She keeps asking if I have a sperm problem and when I say I haven't, she tells me I am a good patient. But it has done my wife the world of good. She hasn't been as well in years even if she isn't pregnant yet.*'

The wife continues: '*During my natural therapy it was discovered I have a thyroid problem, so I have to take thyroxine; my hair was falling out and my nails were breaking. The natural therapist I go to is also a trained counsellor. She told me it takes a good twelve months of natural therapies to prepare you for a pregnancy. It is great to have someone to talk to, she seems to remember your details by heart, whereas the clinic counsellor I see every eight weeks has to look up the details every time, and it hurts.*'

'*My husband came with me to the fertility clinic and asked if there was anything he could do to enhance his health and hence his sperm, and they told him he was fine and not to worry. When we went to the Chinese herbal therapist, she suggested we both go through a cleansing process so we were in synch. It felt good that we were doing something together.*'

Rona Wang is a practitioner of traditional Chinese medicine, trained in Beijing and now working in the Sydney suburb of Leichhardt. She has specialised in gynaecological problems for the past ten years. After a consultation, the patient takes home a bunch of herbs, specifically tailored to their problems. She explained Chinese medicine as an interplay between perpetually contrasting forces of light and dark or yin and yang. A balance between these two forces equals harmony and good health. The aim of the herbalist is to stimulate the yin–yang force and restore balance. One patient recalled her three previous miscarriages and her decision to seek help from Rona:

> There is no denying the herbs taste foul. The liquid looks like mud and smells like rotting seaweed and makes you gag. I had to take a lot of it while I had morning sickness, but it was well worth the effort. I found the best way was to boil down the herbs until I had a real concentrate (and less to drink) then to take a breath in before I swallowed so I couldn't smell the mixture. The minute it was all down, I would bite on an orange or take a teaspoon of marmalade. But I have maintained this pregnancy. Through my pulses, she can now tell me how I am and reassure me as to how my baby is going.

Leonie McMahon advises caution with Chinese herbal medicine. She says there is no doubt that there are good practitioners around and reputable companies producing the herbs. However, she adds:

> Most Australians kick up a stink about drinking the gunk. It is not an attractive therapy, but it can be very effective. I am concerned that many of the naturopaths who take up this therapy are uneducated in pharmacology, and there is no registration on the practice, so you have to be very careful to know that someone is fully trained.
>
> Herbs used in this way are a concentrate, and I do know of a couple of cases who became seriously ill with kidney failure during this therapy. Whatever you do, you have to find someone expertly trained and experienced. With more usual vitamins, the doses are prepared in a laboratory. With homeopathy, you are using dilutions of substances, not concentrates, so there is maximum potential, with minimum product.

Hypnotherapy

Hypnotherapy is often suggested to aid in relaxation, as all investigations and treatments for fertility have a high level of stress. Hypnotherapy is dealt with in detail in the following chapters.

Natural progesterone

Natural progesterone (as opposed to the chemically-produced progestogen) is gaining increasing popularity in the treatment of many problems related to the woman's reproductive system, from PMT to menopause. For people suffering from unexplained or idiopathic infertility, or those who have had recurrent miscarriages, this may provide a natural alternative to more invasive treatments.

Health writer Leslie Kenton, in her book *Passage to Power* (Ebury Press, London, 1995), brought to prominence the work of an American general practitioner or phsyician Dr John Lee, who had been treating his female patients with natural progesterone cream, with great success. Oestrogen has been the hormone high on everyone's agenda in the great hormone replacement therapy revolution which has taken place in the past twenty years. Dr Lee has found natural progesterone to be a more effective therapy.

Progesterone is secreted naturally in our bodies by the corpus luteum, the 'yellow body' that remains in the ovary after ovulation. Progesterone induces the cyclic changes in the endometrium that allow implantation of the fertilised ovum. Progesterone is also responsible for the maintenance of the uterus during pregnancy, suppression of uterine contractions until just prior to parturition (birth) and preparation of the breasts for lactation. (From Aeron Life Cycles pamphlet, *Progesterone and Total Progestins: Quantitative Analysis of Saliva Specimens*)

Dr Lee found that progesterone helps balance the other hormones in the complex bodily system. As well as its role in the preparation of the body for a pregnancy, it has a role of precursor, meaning it is capable of changing into other hormones within the body as they are needed, thus maintaining hormonal balance. Natural progesterone comes from the wild yam. Because it is a natural substance, it cannot be patented, so for drug companies to make large profits from it, they have to alter it to produce a patentable drug. They created progestogen, a synthetic compound which is used within hormone therapies.

It is important to note, however, that although both the synthetic and the natural progesterone can sustain the lining of the womb, the natural hormone can go on to protect a pregnancy from miscarriage. This is not the case with the synthetic version, which carries a warning that it may cause early abortion and birth defects. There is confusion in the two terms *progesterone* and *progestogen*, even with doctors. So the caution which must be applied with the synthetic variation is not necessary with the naturally occurring hormone.

How do you use natural progesterone? In the 1950s, British gynaecologist Dr Katharina Dalton discovered the benefits of progesterone injections for patients suffering from PMT. And she discovered her frequent migraines improved when she was pregnant and producing large amounts of progesterone naturally. Injections, however, can be costly and inconvenient. Later, doctors developed an oral version, but found that once in the stomach it converted into a water-soluble product which is then excreted. After all the experimentation, it has been found that progesterone cream or oil, absorbed transdermally (by the skin), is the most effective form for distribution throughout the body. Vaginal pessaries are also used.

How is it used to enhance fertility? Dr Lee suggests three months of natural progesterone treatment to his patients. He recommends that they use progesterone cream starting on day 10 or 12 of their cycle, before ovulation should take place, until day 28 of her cycle. Then she should stop, and begin counting again when her period comes, counting the first day of her period as day 1. This is done for three months, actually suppressing ovulation. He suggests the woman stop using the cream in the fourth month, assuming the hormonal cycles have become regular, and ovulation will occur at the right time. He has had much success with this method of treatment.

Natural progesterone can also help when progesterone levels drop dramatically after the birth of a baby, creating depression in some women. As it is a natural substance, occurring in different levels in a woman throughout her reproductive life, progesterone presents no dangers.

There may be some mid-cycle spotting initially as the body begins to balance its hormonal systems, and occasionally some breast tenderness again as part of the balancing of the hormonal system. Francesca Naish, in the ACCESS Fact Sheet on natural medicine and infertility, states that:

There is little to lose by choosing to treat infertility naturally, because general health and emotional health should improve. There is benefit from the self-help aspect of many of the therapies, as the patients feel they are active in managing their own recovery.

'Holistic healing accepts that the body, mind and spirit form an integrated whole and that the individual is deeply connected to her environment, her community, and her world. Though we are physically made up of cells, tissues and organs and so on, no parts of us can be understood as isolated entities; all interconnected, they are harmoniously related.'
The New Our Bodies, Ourselves, 25th Anniversary Edition, The Boston Women's Health Book Collective, Simon & Schuster, 1996

Chapter 13
The Fertile Mind

'I always felt that my children were somewhere, I just had to find out how
to bring them into this world. It was like they were trapped in a burning house
and I couldn't get them out through the door. I just had to find another way in and
out to bring them safely to me and my husband. Other times, I used to imagine all
sorts of horrible things. Rather than a mental block I used to figure there was
something wrong that was totally untreatable, like I was born without ovaries
or a womb and no-one was game enough to tell me. Every examination
I used to hold my breath and panic that this was the time they were going
to say there is absolutely nothing that is ever going to help me.'
Mother-of-one, Queensland, Australia

How can we create a fertile environment or does such a thing exist, and why are so
many infertile couples diagnosed as having unexplained infertility? For most people, this
is the hardest diagnosis of all. Somehow, if you know you have a specific problem, the
natural human instinct is to attack the problem and help solve it. Knowing there is no
tangible reason for a pregnancy not to happen, however, causes intense frustration and
a sense of hopelessness. And of course, well-meaning friends bring out all the cliches
such as 'Adopt a baby, people always conceive when they've adopted a baby.' The sheer
ignorance of this comment is insulting, considering there are fewer than 200 babies
available for adoption each year in Britain or Australia, and there are around one in six
couples who suffer a degree of infertility.

'The old story, that if you are infertile, adopt a baby and you'll get pregnant,
statistically we know that just doesn't work,' said Dr Stephen Steigrad. 'Of course stress
is a factor. We don't really know why women conceive in times of war and famine. We
do know stress can stop them ovulating, but we don't know if stress can make them
ovulate badly or inadequately. We don't know how to detect this. We know anxiety in
infertile patients is high. The so-called experts will tell us that stress levels in infertility
patients who actually conceive goes down. Now what a brilliant piece of observation.'

Melbourne professors Carl Wood and Gab Kovacs comment on emotional factors in
infertility:

*Emotional stress may be responsible for causing infertility through the woman
unconsciously avoiding intercourse at the optimal time for becoming pregnant, or
it may cause her to develop fear or pain during intercourse. Anxiety may be
associated with hostile cervical mucus, unreceptive endometrium or tubal spasm.*

In men it may manifest as impotence, premature ejaculation, or impairment of sperm production. These are all hypothetical causes and the mechanism of how they might happen cannot be explained. Studies comparing anxiety levels in infertile couples certainly show it is elevated when compared to fertile couples. On analysing the type of anxiety it appears that it is probably caused by the fertility problems rather than itself being the reason for the subfertility.

From Professor Carl Wood and Professor Gab Kovacs, *Infertility: All Your Questions Answered,* Hill of Content Publishing, 1996

Counsellors attached to clinics are there to allay some of these anxieties. There is no doubt there are good ones. However, because infertility counselling is still a relatively new field, few of the patients interviewed for this book found the counselling they were offered helpful. This will presumably change as the field advances, but most patients reported they found more help and comfort in joining a support group, where they could confide their fears and worries, than with the counsellor attached to their clinic, to whom they felt they couldn't reveal their stress and anxiety, for fear of being taken off the program because they weren't coping.

Clinics vary in the attitudes to counselling. Most have a counsellor attached to their infertility programs; it is mandatory in Australia. Certainly, in most countries people undergoing donor treatment are required to have counselling, to make sure they are aware of the path they have chosen. Professor Robert Jansen of Sydney IVF, Australia, said: 'Sydney IVF is relatively expensive because of high staff:patient ratio, so that there is time for conversation or counselling.'

Paul Entwistle is the director of The Rodney Fertility Clinic, a donor insemination clinic in Liverpool, England. Although a biochemist by training, he has worked in infertility treatment since the 1970s. While dealing with the problems patients faced throughout their treatments, he trained as a counsellor, then as a hypnotherapist, to, as he says, 'make the trying less trying'.

I discovered his work while reading an article in *Good Housekeeping* on a plane journey back to Australia. The article was called 'The Fertile Mind', and discussed his work with hypnotherapy to relieve stress and remove hidden blocks in infertility. Paul Entwistle told how, while working as a scientist in infertility investigation, he had realised other (hidden) factors were also important in achieving a successful pregnancy.

He is one of a small number of counsellors working with hypnotherapy and relaxation, and aside from the more dramatic responses in releasing hidden barriers, he has found beneficial results in most areas, especially with patients diagnosed with unexplained infertility. I found his hypotheses so compelling, they struck a deep chord of truth in me. Six years later, when I started thinking about doing this book, I pulled out the copy of the article, 'The Fertile Mind'. I had photocopied it many times over the years to give to friends in need. I wrote to Paul Entwistle, asking if he'd contribute to the book. I'm grateful he did, as I am sure his experiences and insight will help others, as they did me. I know I have the fertility clinic to thank for putting the good sperm in the right place at the right time. However, recognising I had no vision of myself with a child and re-programming that must have helped, too. He continues to tell us about his work in his own words.

Counselling alone was proving useful in managing infertility and allowing people to continue trying. This may seem an obvious statement, but of course I am going back seventeen years to a time when even talking to patients was slightly unusual. But for many patients, talking alone wasn't enough and I felt I would like to be able to offer a more practical and positive way of helping patients achieve and maintain a greater depth of both physical and emotional relaxation. Among the options I considered were yoga, meditation and tai chi and hypnosis, most of which were not really practical in a clinic situation. Hypnotherapy seemed to be the only real choice.

At that point I had no real experience of hypnosis, though I was a firm believer in the role of the unconscious mind in ruling the body despite being a very formal, scientifically trained biochemist. I therefore set about getting some training in hypnotherapy and had a colleague who had a GP friend in the Midlands, who having retired from the health service, was now running a busy clinic in hypnosis and offered to spend some time training me. So I went down to Leicester and spent some time there working with this GP. I returned to Liverpool and began, very tentatively, to use hypnosis purely for relaxation with some of the patients after DI sessions with some background music I have chosen and which I have always used since, a piece designed for meditation and relaxation.

At that stage I was simply talking to patients, talking them down to a nice deep relaxed state and suggesting that this relaxation and these positive feelings could persist even after they were awake and on their way home, and in the days and weeks following. And it proved successful. Patients did benefit, felt more relaxed and confident and better able to deal with their life outside infertility with their partners and to continue attending for treatment feeling better and more relaxed about the whole thing.

IMPROVED CYCLES

I began to notice that not only were some of these patients more relaxed, but other things about them seemed to improve. Their cycles became more regular, more reliable, measures of hormone action like progesterone and prolactin would often be better in patients who had been receiving the hypnosis and finally, of course, some patients became pregnant after the sessions of hypnosis, though by no means all of them.

Other patients became pregnant during the course of donor insemination combined with hypnotherapy simply because they were able to continue longer in treatment feeling more relaxed and in control. This is, of course, one of the major benefits of counselling and hypnotherapy, because in allowing patients to continue longer they are more likely to achieve a pregnancy.

It is still the case that for every patient achieving a pregnancy, either from natural lovemaking, DI up to ICSI and IVF, it isn't only how well you do what you do in any given cycle, but how many cycles you do it for that determines the likelihood of a pregnancy, a baby and a family. If the treatment can be made more bearable or the lovemaking can be made more stress-free, patients will continue for longer and are far more likely to end with a baby and a family.

There is no doubt that allowing or teaching patients to relax physically and mentally is beneficial to them in the short term and the long term, and also for those patients who didn't conceive and stopped treatment. The benefits for these patients were that they felt they had made the decision to stop treatment in a more relaxed and positive frame of mind, and felt that they had done all that they could possibly do to achieve a pregnancy before giving up — rather than feeling frustrated that they hadn't had a real chance to do it their way. They also moved on to higher tech methods such as IVF and felt better able to try these and work through those because of the positive feelings they had gained with the hypnosis during the DI treatment.

Two features of the use of hypnosis in the DI clinic struck me as being highly significant and going beyond simply the relaxation aspect of what we were doing.

First, there were those women who often quite spectacularly achieved a pregnancy following perhaps just a couple of sessions of hypnotherapy, when many sessions previously of DI alone had been unable to achieve a pregnancy.

Conversely, there were those women who had failed to achieve a pregnancy over a long period of time even with hypnotherapy and despite normal cycles, good hormones and every indication of being fertile. In other words, one group of women became highly fertile just from hypnosis sessions and another group failed totally to become at all fertile from hypnosis or at least hypnosis as I was doing it at that point.

UNEXPLAINED INFERTILITY

The group of patients that attracted my attention were those that had unexplained infertility: either that nothing at all had been found to explain their failure to achieve a pregnancy as a couple or to achieve a pregnancy with the appropriate treatment. Some of those couples or patients had been given a bit of a bad report such as low sperm count or irregular cycles, but I did not feel the reasons given were sufficiently powerful to produce such a high degree of infertility and I regarded some of these as relatively unexplained. I therefore realised that relaxation alone was not enough and that there was more to conceiving than eggs and sperm and tubes and hormones — that there were subtle physical factors controlling fertility which were not detectable by standard investigative approaches.

MECHANISMS

I should perhaps point out my feeling that all subconscious or emotional infertility must ultimately mediate effect through some physical, physiological or biochemical mechanism. Even if the reason for the infertility is in the unconscious mind, there has to be some means whereby an egg is prevented from becoming fertilised, or a fertilised egg is prevented from implanting adequately. You cannot just think a sperm away so that the finding of a physical problem does not preclude an emotional cause for the physical problem. And even in the absence of a measurable physical or physiological problem, if a woman is failing to conceive and yet there is evidence that sperm are going into her body, then there has to be somewhere a means whereby the pregnancy is being physically prevented from commencing or continuing. And that really forms the basis of what I regard as fertility enhancement using hypnosis and hypnotherapy.

I began to suggest to my patients whilst in hypnosis that they became more fertile. In hypnosis, you are talking to the unconscious mind because the conscious mind, the normal centre and filter of incoming signals, has been allowed to drift away. The unconscious mind (in hypnosis) is near the surface and can be talked to in a powerful way. And it is the unconscious mind, not the conscious, that decides when to ovulate and when to have LH (luteinizing hormone) surges and when to signal for hunger. Talking to the unconscious mind is talking directly to the program that runs our bodies.

FERTILITY ENHANCEMENT

The unconscious mind, if it wishes, can improve the physical mechanisms that control and influence conception. So I began to talk to patients under hypnosis about becoming more fertile without specifying exactly what I meant because I do not know what each person's unconscious mind needs to do to make them more fertile. But there is always some room for improvement. This approach I continue to use today. Patients will often in sessions feel some feedback of changes in their bodies, perhaps a warm feeling around their ovaries or uterus which may or may not be effecting a physical enhancement of blood flow, which is certainly the unconscious mind targeting that organ or part of the abdomen which was tense. Very often instructions to become more fertile were reflected in responses in hormone levels with spectacular increases in fertility and pregnancies.

In giving instructions to become more fertile, I always say fertile, not pregnant. Getting pregnant is to a degree out of the control of the unconscious mind, there is a hit and miss, a randomness about egg quality and embryo quality and implantation which means the unconscious mind can never guarantee a pregnancy; it can merely increase fertility to a point where pregnancy becomes highly likely. In asking it to make this person more fertile, I am not thinking clearly of changes in the physical state of the person alone, as I explain to couples.

In order to conceive we need to be in what is seen by the unconscious mind as a fertile environment, fertile for that patient and for them *as a couple* if she has a partner.

Some of the changes that have to take place to make for a fertile situation may be related to interaction between her and her partner, or her and her environment. And often people report changes in the relationship with their partner and others. These changes seem to precede her becoming pregnant. Even when the male partner is totally infertile, I try to encourage him to be involved in what we are doing. His role in making for a fertile relationship is just as powerful in emotional terms as it is for a man with sperm. Him saying the right thing to his partner and making the right noises during the cycle and feeding back in an intuitive way what his partner, the patient, needs to hear, can all reassure her unconscious mind that it is now OK for her to conceive.

For many patients I've seen over the years, I have felt that the female is *holding off* from conceiving because of doubts which she is only barely aware of. About the suitability of her having a child in this relationship — this applies especially to those men who had a previous partnership with children. His new partner may feel uneasy that having left his previous wife or partner, if she were to become pregnant and have children, would he now leave her when she has children also?

Similarly, if she in a previous relationship has had a partner leave her once she became pregnant, or even if she lost it through a miscarriage or termination of pregnancy, the woman needs to be reassured that her present partner would not leave her as her previous one did once she has become pregnant. Even though she knows this at a conscious level, subconsciously, her mind can be holding off getting fertile and pregnant just in case. So that working with a couple even when the man is not contributing in a physical way to the conception, does allow both her conscious mind to explore these reservations and allows the subconscious doubts to surface and be dealt with in a logical and final manner. So the emotional state has to improve first of all and once this has taken place the subconscious mind then allows physical fertility to come about or be enhanced and in due course, hopefully a pregnancy.

SUBCONSCIOUS BARRIERS

The other aspect of how I see the role of hypnosis and hypnotherapy is in exploring subconscious barriers to fertility. As part of working towards that end in my training, I did a series of hypnosis training sessions in Birmingham. The emphasis here was on exploring the unconscious mind through a range of guided images looking for problems and barriers to healing whatever problem — whatever physical problem at least — was preventing fertility.

The sorts of things that set up barriers to fertility are quite small events in the past and are only specifically targeted at fertility. In every other respect, that person is a sane, healthy, well-balanced individual. And only in respect to fertility is there a problem.

There have been several studies by psychologists attempting to show whether couples with infertility have a major emotional problem and they have put such patients through a whole list of psychological tests only to find they are as sane and well-balanced as any other normal individual and therefore have concluded that there is no *emotional factor* in that couple's infertility. But the emotional factors are very specific and will only show in tests which relate to infertility in the same way that it does if you have somebody who has a fear of lifts — perhaps relating to some event in the past as a child trapped in a lift with a barking dog or a nasty person. In every respect, in every test you do on that individual, he will be sane, normal, well-balanced. But if you put him through some questions concerning lifts, you will find the barrier that has to do with lifts.

So if clinicians try to show that there are emotional factors in infertility, they are looking for some dramatic imbalance in that person which they will not find.

PATIENT EXPERIENCES

The following are case histories and some examples of reasons for not conceiving which have then been cured during hypnotherapy. One woman comes to mind — I'll call her Pat. She originally approached me because she was not able to achieve a regular menstrual cycle, never had been, even with all the drugs that were available. She approached me for some emotional help.

In Pat's second hypnotherapy session, she became quite upset and distressed about the fact that her mother, while she was carrying Pat, had become diabetic. This continued after she had delivered Pat to the point where she was having great difficulty dealing with her diabetes. So Pat grew up knowing that her mother had become ill as a result of having her. As Pat was growing up her mother would often comment on this to her friends in front of her, half-joking, but half really getting back at her daughter and Pat took this on board, again half-jokingly and half quite painfully.

In her 30s, Pat thought she had dealt with this and this was no longer a problem, but it came out in that session as being very painful to her. And it would seem that at some point Pat had decided that either she didn't deserve a baby because of what she did to her mother or that she wouldn't have a baby in case what happened to her mother happened to her. In either case, this became a factor in her infertility.

After the second session, she had a very bad week and was quite tearful. She rang me quite concerned and I told her it was OK, as something was coming out. Pat fell pregnant within six weeks, to her amazement. Unfortunately, this was badly handled by her gynaecologist who was very hostile to her having been to me in the first place. And he was actually so hostile and so bullying, I feel this caused her to miscarry at six weeks. She then went on further to have three regular cycles, which hadn't happened before, and then conceived and had a full-term, normal-delivery baby girl. Her periods did not resume after this, so when the time came for a second baby, Pat once more sought my help and we had a long discussion about how we would proceed with further hypnotherapy. Unfortunately or fortunately, the day after that meeting she realised she had ovulated. In that cycle, she conceived again and had her second daughter in due course. Just deciding to discuss therapy was enough to trigger a release of the barrier and helped her to become extremely fertile and to conceive.

The iron gates

Another case was a woman from Ireland who had been trying to achieve a pregnancy for some time, having had three or four failed IVF attempts. At the point that I saw her, she was in her mid-30s, and her story was that when she was living in Ireland and was first married, she decided not to have a baby because she felt there were so many orphan children in Ireland who would be better off being adopted by her than having her own child. This decision destabilised her marriage and she was divorced. She then came to England, remarried and decided she would like to have a baby with her new husband, but she would wait a little while until her career was firmly established before trying for a baby. She in fact waited for about twelve or thirteen years. She then decided now is the time to have a baby and came off the contraceptive pill. She then began trying for a baby, but for a lot of the time her chances were limited by the irregularity of her cycle and loss of libido, to a point that she fairly quickly had to look to IVF because by now she was in her mid- to late-30s. Her attempts at IVF proved unsuccessful for various reasons — she either had a cold prior to her IVF attempt or her cycle the month before became erratic again, or in one cycle she forgot to take two out of the five Clomid tablets, which she found very surprising after all the years she had taken the contraceptive pill and she never once missed one of those tablets.

When she realised what she'd been doing, she admitted to herself that for most of her adult life she'd been avoiding, by some pretext or other, getting pregnant, and there was obviously a very major fertility problem somewhere in her unconscious mind. During some hypnosis sessions, I took her back to childhood and she became upset when we discussed a time when she was five years old — also repeatedly in her sessions she was seeing wrought iron gates. She then went back to Ireland to talk to her parents about her childhood. And it appeared that when she was five years old, her father developed tuberculosis and in those days this was a killer. He was put into a sanatorium and for three years she had no access to him. But she did overhear her mother being told by a doctor that she should not have any more children, the doctor feeling that, as the husband was quite frail, any more children would be a worry to him and also he might not live much longer. Unfortunately the little girl took this to mean that having children makes daddies ill and she was being punished by having her father taken away from her. Even though her father didn't die, by the time he was released from the sanatorium, the little girl had decided that there was a connection between [pregnancy and] daddies becoming ill and possibly dying. And she went back to see the sanatorium where he had been all those years ago, which was now a country house hotel, but they still had the wrought iron gates, which she had seen in hypnotherapy sessions in Liverpool. She had decided to become infertile at five years old.

RELEASING THE BARRIERS THROUGH HYPNOTHERAPY — THE THEORY

Why does hypnosis allow such barriers to be released?

The principle is that the unconscious mind makes decisions on our behalf; it's making them all day in every act we carry out and every result of our actions is monitored by the unconscious mind. In its efforts to determine causality, this can keep us safe and work out the best way first to relate to others and to external situations. In this way, it can plan our future life. And all our actions now are controlled by past decisions made by the unconscious mind. Unfortunately in some situations, the unconscious mind came to an erroneous decision or a decision that was only valid at that time and not for the future. Unless that decision is challenged at some point by the conscious mind, that decision is never chapter-reviewed or updated.

Our conscious minds tend to grow up with us, and change with changing circumstances. But our unconscious minds make very basic decisions which stay with us for the rest of our lives. Thus if as a little girl you were followed home from school on two or three occasions by a tall, bearded man with red hair and you were subsequently warned by your parents to be careful of that man and not to relate to him, then the decision of the unconscious mind to be careful of tall, bearded men with red hair is quite a valid decision at that point in time. However, that decision is put on to your file in the unconscious mind and, even though you have forgotten the episode and the reason for that decision being made, you will continue being uneasy and nervous in the presence of bearded men with red hair.

If one of these happens to be someone with whom you need to relate, like a new boss or your new partner, you will be very ill at ease with that person without knowing why. What has to happen is that the unconscious mind has to tell the conscious mind at some point that this is why you are frightened of bearded men with red hair. And that decision that was made all those years ago can now be modified or updated to allow you to relate to such men in the future.

Alternatively, the unconscious mind can come to a totally erroneous conclusion, because if one event follows closely after another event, then the unconscious mind will make the assumption that the first event caused the second event. If, as a teenager, you become pregnant or even think you've become pregnant, and at the same time somebody close to you becomes ill or your friend's father dies, then the unconscious mind may very well link getting pregnant — particularly if there is a guilt to do with that — with that other person becoming ill or dying. And whenever in the future you choose to get pregnant, the unconscious mind will prevent this knowing, or thinking it knows, that last time you got pregnant your friend became ill or someone died.

The use of hypnosis in these situations is to persuade the unconscious mind to tell the conscious mind why that decision was made. When the unconscious mind comes clean and presents its reasons to the conscious mind, the conscious mind can dismiss those reasons, saying that they are no longer or never were valid reasons and that problem will cease to exist. Obviously, if the reason the unconscious mind made a decision in the past was and still is valid, then the conscious mind will have to accept that and be grateful for the unconscious mind watchdog.

If, for instance, you overheard your parents talking to the family doctor when you were young, and he said he could diagnose in you a very rare condition which meant that if you ever conceived you would become ill and die, then that decision made by your unconscious mind when you overheard the conversation is a very valid decision and should remain in place all your life. If in years to come your parents and doctor all died, your unconscious mind is the only one in possession of that information. Then it has a very valuable job to do in keeping you safe over the rest of your life by inhibiting your fertility. Just as the unconscious mind protects you touching an iron or stepping onto a road because it knows they are dangerous.

If past decisions are still valid, the conscious mind has to accept that. But in practice, there is no real reason why any given person should not become a parent. If their unconscious mind thinks there is, it is wrong. The sooner it tells the conscious mind what the problem is, the sooner the conscious mind can correct that assumption and move on to becoming fertile. That is the principle of searching for these barriers. To correct such decisions made in the past that are inhibiting progress in our lives in the present and future.

SUSPICION ABOUT HYPNOTHERAPY

Some people are naturally wary of hypnosis, particularly with the increasing use of hypnosis as a form of entertainment on the stage, so they often prefer to hear it called relaxation and stress reduction. Often the people I see are those who have approached me formally for hypnotherapy because their infertility is unexplained, either as a couple or as individuals. They feel it is worth trying hypnotherapy or the natural approach with massage and aromatherapy, because they genuinely feel there may be a problem. Perhaps they have had a past history of a pregnancy termination or marital problems, or childhood problems or sexual problems which they feel may be underlying their failure to conceive. And if somebody does approach particularly asking for hypnosis therapy, provided that they are there willingly and not being pushed to me by pressure from their partner or friends and relatives, then it is usually very appropriate to do hypnosis.

COUNSELLING VERSUS HYPNOTHERAPY

Counselling can be less effective than hypnotherapy. The benefits of hypnotherapy are that often patients find it difficult to talk, particularly men. Hypnosis helps this. I also feel that hypnosis can often be faster — one can achieve a lot more in a single session than you can in perhaps several counselling sessions as you are by-passing the conscious mind and going straight to the source of the problem, the unconscious mind — whereas in counselling you have to wait for the unconscious mind to put the words into his or her mouth. Which it does eventually. That can take time, but I often do a mixture of the two and certainly a good counselling technique is forcing the conscious mind to ask the unconscious mind 'What's going on in there? What is happening inside of me?'

But also, counselling does not necessarily achieve relaxation. Neither always does hypnotherapy. If there is a problem from the past — anger, distress, pain — which is now lodged and inhibiting fertility in the present, then searching for and finding that time when the pain occurred will usually trigger that pain again and the patient will re-experience the pain, the anger, the sadness for that bereavement all over again. So I do warn patients that hypnosis sessions are not always totally relaxing or pleasant. But at the start one expects hypnotherapy, as I do it, will bring relaxation and the patient then gets a tape to take away and play at home and it helps him/her to relax.

Counselling isn't specifically designed as a relaxation — it is a discharge of emotions not necessarily designed for physical calm.

Chapter 14
The Status of Surrogacy

'And Sarai said unto Abram, behold now, the Lord hath restrained
me from bearing; I pray thee go in unto my maid: it may be that I may obtain
children by her. And Abram hearkened to the voice of Sarai.'
Genesis 16:2, Old Testament, The Bible

~

'I felt a failure at not being able to get pregnant. Every month I cried
when I had a period, whether on treatment or not. I would get over it after a few
days, but the next month I'd be crying again. That stopped when our surrogate
became pregnant and we have never looked back since.
Successful surrogacy, 1990s

Of all forms of assisted reproduction, surrogacy seems to produce the most outrage from the child-blessed masses. Yet it is the oldest form of fertility aid, quoted in The Bible in Genesis, when Sarai and Abram (re-named by God later as Sarah and Abraham) recruited her maid Hagar to produce Ishmael, Abraham's first son.

Perhaps the fact that this first surrogacy arrangement wasn't successful remains in our genetic memory and produces hysteria when the subject comes up in our times. Hagar reacted to her pregnancy by despising the infertile Sarai, while when the re-christened Sarah and Abraham were blessed by the birth of Isaac in old age, Sarah in turn rejected Ishmael, her husband's first son, and his surrogate mother ... and, as they say, the rest is history.

Some distinctions have to be made between that first surrogacy arrangement to surrogacy in our advanced technological age. These differences are rarely made apparent in sensational media cases, whose endings are not dissimilar to the original flawed emotional contract.

Surrogacy is first divided into two halves—commercial and compassionate surrogacy. In many countries, commercial surrogacy is against the law, and altruistic surrogacy is the only option available to couples where it is impossible for the woman physically to bear a child. In Australia, the United Kingdom and New Zealand, if surrogacy occurs at all, couples are only allowed to pay surrogates reasonable expenses for their maintenance during the pregnancy. In the United States, surrogacy can be carried out by a commercial organisation. The surrogate is usually paid a fee (of around US$10 000 plus expenses). The agent, who may also be a lawyer, gets fees ranging from US$10 000 to $25 000 for arranging the transaction, including the selection and counselling of the surrogate and drawing up the contracts.

Proponents of the United States system claim that, because it is arranged by a commercial agency, it is less likely to go wrong as counselling and selection are more rigorous (one agency in California claims it rejects nineteen out of twenty applicants) and legal contracts are more binding should any of the parties change their minds. Many US state legislatures are debating whether contracts signed before the birth should be legally binding afterwards, should the woman bearing the child change her mind. These agencies also oversee all financial transactions.

The other major area of confusion is the type of surrogacy and whose genetic material is being used. If the egg of the surrogate mother is being used with the commissioning husband's sperm, medical intervention is often not required, although for the surrogate's safety and that of the resulting child, the husband giving the sperm should be tested for HIV and other infectious disease over a six-month period (in the same way men are screened before sperm donations to infertile couples). This is usually referred to as traditional surrogacy. In DIY surrogacy, a simple home-syringe is used and couples organise the inseminations themselves, or other times a gynaecologist will perform the inseminations of the husband's sperm into the surrogate mother during her fertile period.

IVF or host or gestational surrogacy is an entirely different procedure, requiring a lot of medical intervention. As the commissioning mother actually provides her own egg for fertilisation by her husband's sperm in the laboratory, the surrogate mother must have her cycle synchronised with that of the mother, so that when the embryo is ready for transfer, the surrogate's uterine lining is at the right stage in her menstrual cycle to support an embryo. If the embryo has been frozen, synchronisation is not necessary. With IVF surrogacy, the surrogate mother is providing an incubator for the baby, not half the genetic origins of the baby.

From the amount of publicity that explodes if a surrogacy arrangement goes wrong and the birth mother wants to keep the child, it may be assumed that surrogate births are happening all the time, that they are legal and commonplace everywhere, and that they always go wrong. This is not the case.

In Australia, there was a celebrated — and very successful — case where two sisters entered into a surrogacy arrangement. These sisters, Linda and Maggie Kirkman, are in fact one of only two cases of IVF surrogacy to have been reported in Australia. Without national legislation covering reproductive practices, the various state laws make surrogacy a minefield in Australia.

'Surrogacy legislation should be clarified at a national level,' said Professor John Leeton, an IVF pioneer and leading gynaecologist. 'Continuing conflicting legislation effectively restricts couples receiving IVF surrogacy treatments in this country.'

Many couples are forced to make an expensive trip to the United States where commercial agencies organise all aspects of a surrogacy arrangement. An Australian couple was quoted US$45 000 to undertake surrogacy in California using the couple's own embryo and a host or gestational surrogate. When they investigated the situation in Australia, they were told by one New South Wales doctor that such a surrogacy could only be undertaken if a sister or family member acted as the surrogate.

In the United Kingdom, surrogacy is not against the law. However, most clinics require that a couple has failed to conceive through IVF several times to justify host surrogacy. For traditional surrogacy, a hospital or fertility clinic is not necessary. (However, given the risk of HIV or hepatitis infection, perhaps it should be.) COTS or Childlessness Overcome through Surrogacy is a body in the United Kingdom which helps couples organise surrogacy. They have people seeking help from many countries throughout the world, including a recently publicised case of a couple from the Netherlands and their dispute with the woman who was bearing a child for them, conceived using the husband's sperm. Initially, the surrogate claimed she'd had the child aborted, but then admitted she and her husband had agreed to make the child part of their own family. The acrimony between the surrogate and commissioning couple was tabloid media fodder and resulted in a British government inquiry into the whole issue of surrogacy. Kim Cotton, head of COTS, the altruistic surrogacy group who introduced the two parties, argued that because theirs is a voluntary group, they do not have the time nor the money to spend on rigorous counselling and legal work to avoid these situations. She also states that of the 200 births her organisation has coordinated, you could count on the fingers of one hand the number that have become human tragedies.

In Australia, a law has been passed in the Australian Capital Territory (ACT) called the *Substitute Parents Agreements (Consequential Amendments) Act 1994*. The act is still unclear about the legal outcome relating to the child, and further amendments must be made. An IVF surrogacy is yet to be carried out in the ACT to test this law.

It is now nine years since the Kirkman sisters gave birth to Alice. As they were very close, many of the emotional implications about bearing and giving up a child do not apply in their case. Linda, the host mother, has a natural role as Alice's aunt — a very special

SURROGACY AND THE LAW

Legal complexities within surrogacy abound — many because of laws introduced to protect children born of donated sperm, eggs or embryos. In most countries, when the child is born from conception with donated sperm, the legal father is the male partner and the child is regarded as the child of that partnership. The same applies when a woman gives birth to a child using donated eggs or a donated embryo. The child's mother is designated as the woman who gestated and bore that child.

In surrogacy, the reverse needs to apply in both cases. By the previous law, the legal father of the child would be the partner of the woman bearing that child — the surrogate — not the commissioning male partner, whose semen was used to create the child. Also, because of the law designed to protect children of donor eggs or embryos, the legal mother of a child born to a surrogate is the surrogate, as she is the one to gestate and carry the child.

Hence, a law designed to protect one group using assisted reproductive technology actually thwarts others, requiring legal adoption by the commissioning couple, as explained later in this chapter.

aunt. Maggie, Alice's mother, has said: 'Because she has a continuing relationship with the woman who gestated her, Alice knows she was not merely given away. Linda was not left wondering what became of the baby she bore; she is not grieving over a lost child.'

Linda continued to express breast milk for Maggie to feed Alice for her first four months, and Maggie was able to induce lactation herself during this period. Other women also donated breast milk so this child would have the best start possible.

Alice, now old enough to comment on the situation, simply says, 'I am glad that I am alive and I am lucky to be alive.'

The intimate acts such as breastfeeding a child and who would carry it out would not have been a consideration in centuries past when wet nurses were the order of the day for prosperous families. Now, however, it is seen as part of the mystical bond between mother and child.

One American woman wrote of her decision not to proceed with a surrogate arrangement when the surrogate mother began talking of suckling the subsequent child or children:

A friend of proven fertility offered to try to carry my embryos for me. It is one of those offers that transcends love. But in an offhand moment she says ebulliently, 'I'll breastfeed them too for a few days just to get them started,' and something inside me tenses despite the overwhelming generosity of her offer. My babies, you will breastfeed my babies? And in that instant I have a sharp inkling of how fine the lines are in all this talk of scrambled eggs and borrowed wombs.
Motherhood Deferred: A Woman's Journey, Putnam's Sons, © 1994 Anne Taylor Fleming

Throughout all the emotive talk about what is profit and what are expenses — one morally acceptable in some countries, the other not — plus the complex legislation and the media hype, people forget that there are infertile couples at the centre of it, wanting to start a family.

Surrogacy arrangements can work. It is not a treatment often needed, in fact in Australia, doctors say only about fifty couples per year would require IVF surrogacy. In the absence of clear legal guidelines, surrogacy is often restricted at a medical committee level rather than in a definite statement of law. The success stories are the ones you don't see sensationalised on television or in newspapers. The people simply live their lives with their precious addition to their family.

Jayne and Mark tell the story of their surrogacy arrangement in the United Kingdom, proving it can work, and with joyful results. It is an inspiration to those who seek surrogacy as their only chance to have a child. Jayne tells their story.

For more than ten years, Mark and I tried for a family before surrogacy. We had more than thirty cycles of differing treatments ranging from Clomid to IVF, each in turn failing. The pain of childlessness is hard to imagine for those who have never experienced it. Each month you are reminded of your infertility by your period. No matter how hard you try to forget your desire for a family, you just can't. Everyone asks when you are going to start a family, which is yet another reminder. People who had never experienced infertility would tell me just to relax *and have a bottle of wine. I would tell them I had a fertility problem, not a sexual problem! No amount of relaxing was going to make me ovulate without drugs or thicken my womb lining. Over the years we had many holidays and romantic meals to aid our fertility, all to no avail.*

During our years of infertility, many friends and relatives became pregnant. I was always the first to congratulate them and would be all smiles when I was told of their good news, but I would then cry in private. When was it going to be my turn? What had I done to deserve this?

Many people assured us over the years that being parents was no big deal. Many even wished they could be me if they had their time again, they said they wouldn't have any children. How I wished to be in their shoes! Even a counsellor couldn't understand why I wanted a baby so much and more or less said if she was me she would just give up and enjoy life child free. She had her children, so she couldn't begin to understand how I felt.

After seven years of failed fertility treatment my husband and I decided enough was enough, it was time to move on. As we still wanted children, we decided to apply to adopt. We hoped to be approved as adoptive parents for up to three children, up to the age of five years. As most people seemed to want to adopt babies, we thought we had a good chance. We went through a long and intensive assessment. During our years of infertility, we had built up a nice home and we were quite shocked to find this was to count against us. In our first report it was noted that this had implications on the type of children we could adopt.

Our period of assessment lasted for over two years. A social worker would come every two to three weeks. We felt emotionally drained at the end of it. The last straw came when I informed our social worker that my mother was terminally ill with cancer. We were then told this, too, had implications on our adoption application. We would have to grieve for a year after mum's death before we could be considered. We continued with the adoption thinking we would probably be turned down as our social worker was very negative about us being approved as adoptive parents. At the same time we began to look into surrogacy.

We contacted COTS in May 1995. Within just a few weeks of applying, the secretary at COTS phoned us to say they had a potential surrogate for us. We couldn't believe it as we had expected to wait many months. I phoned Lynne, our surrogate-to-be, and arranged for Mark and I to meet her. We had the choice of traditional surrogacy or IVF surrogacy, but chose the traditional one using the surrogate's egg and my husband's sperm. We didn't feel the need for our child to be genetically related to both of us. I had only one failed attempt at IVF, so most clinics would have told us we hadn't failed enough to justify host surrogacy. After getting to know Lynne, we started our inseminations. COTS provided us with a

DIY insemination kit. It took six cycles to conceive. On 15 February 1996, Lynne phoned to say she was pregnant. We were thrilled. Two days later our social worker called round to say we had also been approved for adoption. We were told it was not a majority decision and that we were lucky to be approved. The panel had approved us for one child under the age of four years. As there are very few children of that age to be adopted we knew it would be unlikely we would be placed with a child in the near future.

When Lynne was 20 weeks pregnant, we told social services that we were expecting a baby and asked for our names to be removed from the waiting list.

At 12 weeks pregnant we had the first scan. It was a wonderful feeling to see our baby waving back at us. We had two further scans throughout the pregnancy because the hospital thought the baby was a little on the small size. The pregnancy had no real problems except for a scare at 32 weeks when Lynne had an ante-natal check and the heartbeat was very slow. We had to wait 24 hours for a detailed scan to check everything was alright. The baby had been asleep which was why the heartbeat was slow. We were all very relieved.

Finally, the day came when Abigail Lynne was to be born. At 11.40 a.m. on 10 October, Lynne phoned to say her waters had broken. She told us to drive carefully as her contractions hadn't started and there was plenty of time for us to get to the hospital. We arrived just after 2 p.m. By now Lynne had started to have contractions, but they stopped as we arrived. We stayed at the hospital with Lynne until about 6 p.m. and as nothing further was happening we went to get something to eat. We went to Lynne's mum's house to await any further news. At about 11.40 p.m. the hospital rang to say we should come over as Lynne was now in labour.

We arrived at about 12.30 a.m. I was allowed into the labour room with Lynne and the midwife. Mark preferred to wait outside as he feels faint just watching 'Casualty' on TV. Lynne had originally opted for a natural birth, but soon changed her mind and had an epidural. At 1.44 a.m., our beautiful daughter was born. Lynne asked if I would like to cut the cord, which I did, then Abigail was handed straight to me.

Meanwhile Mark was pacing up and down outside wondering what was happening. When the baby was cleaned, Mark was invited into the room. He held our daughter and marvelled at her, then we handed her to Lynne to hold while lots of photos were taken. The hospital was wonderful. After the birth, Lynne was given her own room and they also provided a family room for Abigail, Mark and me. A nurse bathed our baby and then we both took it in turn to feed her.

Abigail slept very well and in the morning Lynne's mum came to the hospital to take her home. Before they left Lynne's mum and her children visited Abigail and more photos were taken. We left the hospital in the early afternoon after being given some classes in parenthood, being taught how to bath the baby and make up her bottles. The hospital informed our doctor that we were bringing our baby home and a few days later a midwife visited. From then on, we were treated the same as any new parents. All the medical staff we met have been very supportive throughout and see our baby's birth as being extra special.

After the birth we had to contact the local magistrates court and apply for a 'parental order'. We were able to do this six weeks after the birth. It must be applied for within six months of the birth. This is a special order to legalise us as the parents of our child and was introduced in November 1994 specifically for surrogate children. A parental order is necessary even if you use your own embryo. Previous to this couples had to go through the adoption process. We telephoned the court for the relevant forms, filled them in (they were brief, just requiring our names and address and that of our surrogate mother). We were invited to the court and were asked to prepare a statement for the court explaining our fertility problem and detailing the treatment we'd had. We also had to justify the expenses paid to our surrogate mother. At this meeting we were introduced to a 'Guardian Ad Litem' — a social worker who was looking after Abigail's interests. She wrote a short report about us and visited us twice in order to do this and also visited our surrogate mother. We then had a second hearing at the court. Our evidence and statements were presented to the court and five minutes later we were granted our parental order. Abigail is now legally our child. This order was granted when Abigail was 20 weeks old. She is a wonderful, happy baby. My heart melts whenever she smiles at me. All those years of infertility and hoping are now firmly in the past. I am making the most of every day and enjoying every minute. Motherhood is everything I expected it to be.

I speak on the phone to Lynne, our surrogate mother, every two weeks or so, and we see each other every couple of months. I don't feel threatened by her and she doesn't interfere in the way I bring up Abigail. When she holds Abigail, I can see the joy in her face at bringing such a wanted baby into the world who is so loved by her parents. All Lynne expected from us initially was news on how Abigail was growing up and pictures about once a year. We have become such good friends over the last few months that we see as much of her as we see our other good friends. Lynne also wants to help us have a brother or sister for Abigail next year. Some people are surprised that we still see Lynne. Why not? She is a good friend and always will be.

Abigail will be told how she was born and who her birth mother is as she grows up. We have taken many videos of our meetings with Lynne and her family and intend to show Abigail the videos to help her understand how she was brought into the world. She will be told Lynne carried her in her tummy because I have a broken tummy. When she is old enough to understand about genetics, she will then be told that Lynne also provided her egg and that Lynne's children are her biological half-brother and sister.

Lynne's children understand that Abigail is a special baby and are very proud of their mum for helping us. I am sure Abigail will feel the same when she grows up. We talked about how we would tell our child about her birth before entering the surrogacy arrangement. Our surrogacy organisation won't help couples who are not prepared to tell the child as the child may have an identity crisis if he or she find out too late in life.

When people talk about who she looks like, I don't mind if they say she looks like my husband. I often say I think she looks like our surrogate's daughter too, because she does.

I can't thank Lynne enough for what she has done for us. She has made our lives have substance and meaning. Every day is wonderful now that we have our much-wanted baby. We are a family at last. Our long wait has been worth it. I try and look on the positive side of infertility and think it will make us better parents rather than feeling sad about the lost years and heartache we endured.

If I miraculously conceived naturally in the future that would be OK, but if I returned to treatment and it worked our daughter may think we were not happy with her and feel less loved than the genetic child. This is why adoption agencies insist couples give up treatment once they adopt and I believe this is for a very good reason. Hopefully in the future Abigail will have a brother or sister who will have been brought into the world the same way.

WHAT THE WORLD THINKS AND DOES ABOUT SURROGACY

The New Zealand Infertility Society Incorporated produced a newsletter devoted to the issue of surrogacy. The following summing up of world and religious attitudes is published with their permission.

NEW ZEALAND

In New Zealand, there is still no specific legislation covering surrogacy, although committees have been formed to formulate principles. Recommendations to date call for some sort of regulation, and that there should not be a blanket ban on surrogacy. It recommended that counselling should be available, that parents tell children of their genetic origins, that information should be kept in a similar way to adoption, and consent be comprehensive.

AUSTRALIA

Although the National Bioethics Consultative Committee recommended that surrogacy be allowed, the Health and Social Welfare Ministers made a joint decision to prohibit surrogacy. This decision has not been ratified by law in all states, but the decision has effectively stopped clinics from providing treatment. In Queensland, surrogacy is a criminal offence.

United Kingdom

The *Surrogacy Act of 1985* outlawed commercial surrogacy agencies. The *Human Fertilisation and Embryology Act of 1990* defined the surrogate mother as the mother by law. The parents, with the consent from the surrogate, can apply for a court order to make them the legal parents. The government is now compiling a report on surrogacy in the UK.

UNITED STATES OF AMERICA

The situation varies between states, with eighteen states having laws addressing surrogacy. There are laws in several states that provide guidelines for judges called to decide on custody suits.

A review by the Health Department of New York State estimated 4000 surrogate births since 1970, with eleven reported custody suits. In ten, the child was awarded to the intended parents.

THE NETHERLANDS

It is forbidden to perform embryo transfer to a woman not willing to be the prospective mother. Nevertheless, such treatments have been carried out openly, without legal repercussions.

DENMARK

Commercial aspects of surrogacy are forbidden.

SPAIN

No contract that provides for gestation, with or without payment, by a woman who renounces her maternal bonds in favour of the contractor, or of a third party, shall have any legal validity whatsoever (from *Focus Reprod* 1(4):16 1991).

GERMANY

Oocyte and embryo donation are both forbidden, as is surrogate motherhood (*Focus Reprod* 1(3):7 1991).

NORWAY

Donation of human oocytes is forbidden, thus ruling out surrogacy (*Focus Reprod* 2(1):16, 1992).

FRANCE

The same law applies as in Norway, encouraging 'medical tourism' for couples requiring donor eggs or surrogacy.

ISRAEL

The practice of surrogate motherhood, partial or complete, is forbidden under a 1987 law (*Focus Reprod* 3(1):16, 1993). However, following an appeal, the Supreme Court decided IVF surrogacy may be performed as long as the embryos are transferred to the surrogate outside the state of Israel. It also directed the Ministries of Health and Justice to prepare legislation for the legalisation of surrogacy in Israel.

RELIGIOUS VIEWS

CHRISTIANITY

Surrogate motherhood is not accepted, because it is contrary to the unity of marriage.

JUDAISM

In traditional surrogacy (where the surrogate provides the egg or oocyte), the resulting child belongs to the provider of the sperm. Where IVF or host surrogacy is used, the status of the child is unresolved.

ISLAM

Insemination of the surrogate is considered adultery.

BUDDHISM

Unmarried and married people can seek surrogacy, but it may raise problems with family ties.

HINDUISM

Like Buddhism, there are no prohibitions, but possible dilemmas about family ties, and legal and moral issues could ensue.

CULTURAL PERSPECTIVE

The Maori and Pacific Islanders' attitude is much more compassionate towards the infertile — they are regarded as part of the community with a valuable contribution to make in the raising of a child. Sometimes a child is produced especially for them by another member of the family; often they act as parents to a child or children from a close relative.

Chapter 15
Life after Infertility — An Uncertain Miracle

'I wonder if I was really meant to have a baby, or did I force it? I ask myself
is having a baby everyone's right, or is it somehow a blessing. Five years ago I would
have insisted it was everyone's right. We are such a consumer society, wanting
everything. It's something most of us take for granted and shouldn't.'

What happens after infertility — do we all live happily ever after, content either that we
have managed to have our precious children, or that we have given up after exhausting
the creativity of reproductive science? What do we do with all the emotion and
cumulative experiences, do we let them slip away? Do they automatically recede like the
pain of childbirth? Are we the perfect parents we'd imagined we would be and is our
child the equally perfect reward for all the suffering we went through? Do we dare to
complain about the sleepless nights? Life after infertility is easy for some, not so easy for
others. Some people ease into their roles as parents, grateful and happy to let those
painful memories of infertility fade. For those who have used donor sperm or egg, their
infertility is ever-present, as they make the choices about if and when to tell the child,
how best to assure and reassure themselves, their partner and their child. Or how best
to maintain the secret, if that is their choice.

Many people agree that a child isn't the cure for infertility. Those suffering with
infertility are still infertile. And if they want to add to their family, they have to
contemplate the same procedures as they did for their first child. And if we don't adapt
to maternal or paternal roles easily, what then? What do we do with the guilt feelings
that overpower us?

I look back on those first few years of motherhood with some dismay. Not for our
son, as I put his needs above everything. However, the shock of having a small child erupt
into our adult lives was something I hadn't imagined. I was used to responsibility — for
my staff, of whom I was enormously fond, for financial matters on the magazine — but
this kind of responsibility was entirely different. Here was a small being I couldn't take
my eyes off for one minute, especially once he was crawling. And as a professional used
to achieving things, to know I wasn't going to finish a single independent task, no matter
how mundane, took a huge adjustment.

Of course, other mature parents experience this, too, but at least they feel they can
complain to one and all about this disruption in their lives. When you have really
invested your life in the successful birth of a child, however, you don't dare complain to

anyone if you are not coping — not even your partner. And he probably has the same problem. The complex feelings leading up to the birth don't go away.

Recently, I found I had a strange non-period, then my breasts grew larger, I felt sick — all the signs of a pregnancy. As I was writing the section on egg age at the time, I didn't get excited about this unexpected blessing, knowing with our history, plus the passage of time, a successful pregnancy wouldn't be likely. I reached for the thermometer and also drew up a temperature chart *just to see* what was happening and if my hormone levels were pregnancy-high. It was Christmas and my doctor was away and I kept reminding myself that, at 47, it shouldn't be possible. But again I found myself seduced by the temperature chart, fascinated each morning to know if the levels stayed high. The temperature stayed up for two weeks, and for two weeks I was pitched right back to infertility. I was looking for symptoms, looking for spots on my knickers, pleased and amused when my husband noticed for himself that my breasts had changed.

It didn't last and, with a lot of pain and bleeding, at what would have been six weeks pregnant, it all came away before I had a pregnancy test. The emotions were different this time as it was an unexpected event, and one that had little chance of success. The shattering reality, however, was that I was right back where I'd been prior to our son's birth. Nothing had really changed.

It led me to think that for me, the issue of infertility and fertility will not be finally settled until I am well past menopause. Perhaps then there will be some kind of resolution and peace. Others share their thoughts:

'I still feel I have an infertility problem. I don't feel it is fixed by the birth of a child or even achieving a pregnancy. Because this problem still exists, there are still limits on my choices that would not be there if I was fertile. For example, the choice to try for a second child is in some respects harder than trying for the first. When I went to a psychiatrist to discuss my antagonism to my brother's pregnancy, I asked him what would happen to all the bad feelings I had as a result of infertility if I was to have a baby. He said they would fade and the intensity would go, but I would still remember them. I cannot say our infertility has been solved by the birth of our son. It has masked many of the issues and emotions, and I am grateful he is here with us and realise we may well have not been so lucky. However, the other side is, he is unlikely ever to have brothers and sisters, nieces and nephews. We would have liked a larger family, but given how long it has taken us to have this child, and the emotional cost involved, it is unlikely we will return for further treatment. We are also scared we might not be as lucky next time as we feel our ages are now becoming factors. Not that we want a perfect child, but that our ages are a consideration as to how well we do as parents, not so much with babies, but as kids get older and need active parents.'

~

'I suppose in the back of my mind I had always felt I would not have my own baby — a part of my nothing nice ever happens to me syndrome. I don't feel I can

say to close people like my mum, "She was a little swine today I'm fed up with her." They may say, or think, "Well, you wanted her, you had this special treatment to have her,"' said one woman from England.

Her husband comments: 'We know that she is our only chance, unless we suddenly became very rich, which is unlikely.' [They had to have private treatment to have their child.]

An ordained minister of religion talks about the issues he has faced, some of them not in tune with the teachings of his church:

Infertility is a death experience. The pain of infertility is similar to the stages of dying, as outlined in Elizabeth Kubler-Ross's book On Death and Dying. *This was a part of my journey. If you are unfamiliar with them, they are: (1) denial and isolation, (2) anger, (3) bargaining, (4) depression, (5) acceptance. When you find you cannot achieve a pregnancy and eventually find out you can't father a child, these children (of your hopes) die. You mourn their passing, even though they were never born. My personal feeling at my diagnosis was guilt and shame. I felt a failure. I feared my wife would leave me. I felt that I'd failed my father as I am his only son and his name would die with me, as here ended the genetic line.*

The impression we got from the specialist treating us was that male infertility doesn't really matter. You can always have donor insemination. You'll get your baby. Let me tell you a baby is not a cure for infertility. We have our two beautiful children, but it hasn't changed the fact of my infertility one little bit. At that stage I was very anti-DI. I wasn't ready for it. I still had too much on my plate to sort out. My wife, being a more open person than I, was favourable to the suggestion. I was not. Over the next twelve months, I took my infertility out on her. If I couldn't have a baby, neither could she. If I had to suffer, she had to suffer with me. I found other justifiable arguments such as I didn't want a child fathered THAT way, and besides, the church opposes it. I stuck to those arguments for a number of years.

A colleague in England shares her feelings in the following story. After the initial jubilation after her son's birth two years ago, she developed severe post-natal depression. She has been exploring her reactions as she slowly recovers. Perhaps her thoughts and feelings are not uncommon in fertility survivors. When you focus so much of yourself on to having a child, you invariably neglect other aspects of your life. These issues still have to be dealt with after the treatment stops. You still have to decide where you want to live, where you want to work, what new steps should be taken in your career or if you should stop working and be with your child. And your relationships with your partner, family and friends — any difficulties that have been postponed there still exist.

For me, the emotional issues of infertility recur when you least expect them. I think I was in a kind of trance for the first few years after our son's birth. Everything (except things to do with him) was done on automatic pilot. I look now at some of the clothes

LIFE AFTER INFERTILITY

We had eight years of unexplained infertility. I was 30 and I was a crew member of an airline. There was a trip somewhere, I can't remember, but it was somewhere none of the crew wanted to go — it was a bit dangerous, so I said, 'OK I'll get pregnant.' Up until I decided to have a child, I was pretty hedonistic. My husband is from a kibbutz in Israel, a very strict upbringing, the first son. Leaving the kibbutz for big, bad me was a strong guilt trip for both of us.

When my flying schedule took me to Israel, I would nip out to the kibbutz for a few days and my mother-in-law would be there. She would ask me about having children and I would say something like, 'Oh, I don't need children.' I was having fun. I would love to play back that scene. Pregnancy didn't happen and this continued for some time, and I was flying in different time zones which didn't help my cycles. Then eventually we went for tests, we were sort of playing at it, though you don't realise it at the time.

At the start, treatment was very disjointed — go and have a blood test at the blood bank, go and have the sperm analysed — and later on when we went to a clinic, it was much more specialised, much better. They found out basically that I had unexplained infertility. I was told that I should have a try at IVF, but there was no money on the National Health Service and that we'd have to go for private treatment.

We hadn't grown up with any illnesses, with doctors and hospitals, so we took them at their word and we did try IVF — it didn't work. We had what they call a chemical pregnancy that started to implant then came away and that was pretty traumatic. We were both working and we hadn't told many people.

I went to see a homeopath to try to balance out my hormones, my periods were very painful. She did this, but it meant taking on a lot of changes — in diet, particularly. I don't know if that helped or not but it certainly couldn't do any harm, and it did take away the pain from my periods, which is what I wanted, but you have to work with it.

At about that time I changed my job and worked on a project about cultural awareness between England and Israel — it was good work and it enabled me to work around my treatment — and so it's kind of mixing infertility with your lifestyle. I finally left the airline because by that time, although my job was great, it was very stressful. I made the decision and I worked locally so I could be nearer for treatment. They didn't know about my infertility. And that was difficult, a different working environment, not so dynamic. I went to the local hospital which wasn't very good, but I tried whatever they could offer — IUI (intra-uterine insemination), done by volunteers. After being advised to try IVF, we checked out a couple of people and decided to go to the Hammersmith Hospital because of Professor Winston, the best-known fertility specialist in Britain. Also, because they were a research group and that appealed to us because we had unexplained infertility.

I wasn't into having the drugs. Initially I was quite appalled at it. But I think two years later, and still no baby, I'd become that much more desperate. Not only that, you go and see the specialist/consultant and you accept everything they say — we live in that kind of culture where if the doctor says it, it must be right.

So we became patients at the Hammersmith Hospital and both our parents contributed towards the costs and it was a nice clinic, a bit like a club really. You kind of got used to putting things in your mouth, having things put up your bottom, but I think you underestimate the impact of that at the time.

You are out of control emotionally, because you are just driven by something in you that can't be rationalised. I was most of the time in tears about it, talking about it, everything related to it. The clinic became quite an integral part of our lives, and the people at the clinic. It was nice to be attached to somewhere you could go, with people to ask questions of. They were very supportive and I had counselling at the same time, nothing to do with infertility, and we talked over a lot of issues, then I got pregnant naturally some months after the IVF and I miscarried at 12 weeks so that was pretty devastating.

The clinic was really good giving me scans without charging anything and they were very supportive. They seemed pleased that we had had some sort of result.

We went back to see Professor Winston and he suggested another IVF cycle and I told him I wasn't sure I could go through another one. I was reaching the end — we all have different levels of tolerance. (I do wonder sometimes about the effects of the drugs in IVF. There's no limit to the number of cycles you can have; it's what you can afford. That's why I think people should think about it a little bit more before they choose their course of action. I certainly wouldn't have any more of that kind of treatment.)

Basically I got pregnant again naturally and miscarried — I think it was three miscarriages I had in the end — and they referred us to Recurrent Miscarriage Association. When I went to the Recurrent Miscarriage Clinic, they tested me for various things and said I had normal fertility. After eight infertile years I found that pretty interesting. Each miscarriage was slightly earlier, but basically your life is on hold, you can't do this and you can't do that and any help you are getting you are paying for through the clinic. There was nothing locally, which would have been a lot easier. When you're in pain like that, you need things around you to support you and help you, not things to cause you more stress. And with infertility in this country, unless you pay for it, or you're lucky enough to get that support from your family and friends, there is not much available. The finances are a big issue.

I was the main breadwinner so it was a big pressure on us. I was earning a good salary and then I cut that in half when I left and have gone down since. There are priorities and you make those choices. I didn't have any counselling after my miscarriages. It all came out a bit later with me. I'd left the local job as it was driving me nuts and it was a different kind of working environment. But I was so frustrated inside I couldn't really get into it, so another job came up and I did that—marketing for a private aviation company — I did that job for six months then I had a miscarriage, then I went to work for a large Asian airline, in a supervisory position, looking after the crew. In this company, no one talked or showed emotions, and as I had two miscarriages while I was working there, I finally decided I'd had enough.

My husband took a sabbatical and we were going off round the world. I was on overload, I couldn't take any more. Within a month I was pregnant naturally. I just took the stress out and gave up, and that's how it happened. Coupled with things I was doing with the homeopath, it took me well into the complementary medicine side. I think homeopathy is so beneficial, because you do look at the whole picture.

And there's a reason — the unexplained infertility that these experts say is unexplained — I believe it is explainable. It is just outside their remit, they have one answer to a range of problems and with women I believe there are lots of psychological and emotional issues that cannot be solved with chemicals.

The good doctors will admit that there is a lot they can't explain. But not all of them will. What I have learnt from my own pain has turned things around a bit. There is a lot of resistance to alternative or complementary treatment.

Anyway, after I was pregnant with our son, they monitored me, which was very good, every week for twelve weeks, gave me some added progesterone, and then we went to Israel for four months, which was great. I was going to have the baby out there, but I visited the local hospital and decided against it. I wanted to stay there because we did have the whole year off and it's a lovely environment. Anyway we came back here and he was two weeks early and I had a caesarean, which was fine, and we were really just pleased that he came out alright — I got really anxious.

We were high as two kites and it was great and then I sort of went into huge post-natal depression. I can't remember exactly when, I guess it would have been about eight months after his birth. I think it was a kick-back from all the things we'd been going through, all the anxiety. Fortunately, I went to see my family and my mum got out an article about post-natal depression or something similar and I read it. I wasn't up to doing very much at all. And then, I suppose because I'd learned coping mechanisms within the infertility, I didn't have any hang-ups about saying I wanted some help. And slowly, step by step, I got better.

At the same time, I started to understand what had happened and why it had happened. And then about a year ago, I learned about a natural healer, and that was the right thing at the right time. Someone put me onto her, she has been doing healing for thirty-eight years. I rang her up and told her how I felt and she suggested my hormones might be out of balance, and said, 'That's OK, we can put that right in a couple of weeks.' I thought, Oh yes, sure. And natural healing makes so many connections, why we are infertile, where it is coming from and how we can put it right in a positive way. You've got to dig right into the core of yourself.

There was no history of infertility in our family, no reason for me to be infertile, other than that I was in a job and an environment which wasn't conducive to having children. I think it was a combination of the stress and the fear, but I didn't realise it at the time. Up until dealing with infertility, I was always very outgoing and positive, and then when you come across this, slowly, over a period of years, you change. You get so used to the failure and disappointment that you start losing your identity. My parents said to me this summer, 'You used to be so lively and fun-loving, and now you are so intense.' They don't quite understand, I don't know that I understand. I kind of miss the laughter, because laughter is so therapeutic.

I feel ever since I had my son I've been in a state of anxiety about something and I've never really sat down and just played with him without thinking of the house, the washing, the ironing, work. I need quiet and silence with him and I'm taking it now. I think I need to leave the emotional issues of infertility behind me, I feel the weight is too much and being still involved is not allowing me to move on. Trying for another baby recently brought all the issues back. It was obviously too soon. I don't know if infertility is more prevalent now in the Western world, but if it is, it might just be because the kind of world we are bringing them into isn't conducive to children. When I think of all the warmth and affection on the kibbutz, it makes me think we should move there to bring up our son. Then I think about the bombs ...

I bought then and can't believe it — they were just not like me at all. I accept not all of that has to do with post-infertility. I also left my job and changed countries, all very unsettling. However, as someone who always wanted to achieve the absolute best at work, I switched to trying to do the absolute best by my child. So I did everything for him. He never needed to call out for anything; it was there before he needed it.

My need to give him everything emotionally was overwhelming, too. So it was a shock, after three happy years at infant school, that he was having immense problems in the first year of primary school. The French system is very strict, and the children do go from being babies to small adults in a swift leap. While the others were coping, however, my over-nurtured darling couldn't cope. He had never had to do anything for himself and now he resisted learning. And when these things were demanded of him he was mute with shock that he had to do things for himself.

When the teacher asked if he dressed himself, I confessed he didn't — after all, it was a joy to do these things for my much-wanted child. I savoured every moment of caring for him. Yet, in doing so, I was depriving him of his basic survival skills — and I had to gradually make him take responsibility for himself. A continuing process.

I learned a lesson from the school experience, having to force my child into reluctant autonomy. I assume if I hadn't had problems, I wouldn't have left work, so I wouldn't have had time to cosset him. Then the other part of me says he would be a different person now if he had had to fend for himself in a big nursery, seeing us only briefly in the evenings before bed. I railed against the school system and told them in appalling French that my theory was that too many men never had enough mothering — and still needed it into old age. I felt that if my son was given enough mothering until he stopped needing it, maybe he would end up a complete person.

While a lot of that remains true for me, I do realise some males do need a little kick towards independence, including this little one. My only regret now is that I didn't launch into having another child immediately. At the time, physically and mentally, it was the last thing on my mind. I think, deep down, I felt I was so lucky to have this one, I shouldn't push it. Now I think it was selfish to our son not to try. If I had, he wouldn't be quite so much the centre of the universe. Also, the fears with an only child are very real, even though intellectually you know each would be just as precious if you had two and lost one. One child can't replace another. But when you know this one is IT — the first and only child possible for you — you have to fight constantly against being overprotective, trying all the time not to let it show.

I remember a time when he was a toddler, following him across Centennial Park in Sydney, talking to a friend. We suddenly looked up and he was nowhere to be seen. She said she will never forget the look on my face. I ran in one direction, she the other. It was like one of those awful news stories you see about a child disappearing in a second. After about five frantic minutes, I heard a familiar chuckling. He had somehow climbed the stairs into a little playhouse, and was too small to be seen above the wall!

This burden of fear must never be placed on the child, but the effort to control it is huge. Also, as older parents, I think it was selfish that we didn't think that in the future our child deserved us trying for a sibling for him. A brother or sister, nieces and nephews. He will just have to settle for his adult half-brother and cousins. I am comforted that his cousins all wish they were only children, not a family of four. Life after infertility is an uncertain — and imperfect — miracle. But nevertheless, it *is* a miracle.

Residual Impact of Fertility Drugs

I asked Professor Carl Wood about residual effects of IVF drugs. He replied:

The residual effects of the drugs have been checked out by our own research in Australia, reported in the Lancet *last year. Ten thousand women who had suffered cancer of the breast or ovary were checked for background factors which may increase their chance of developing such cancers. The risk of cancer was not associated with infertility treatment, the use of drugs in tablet or injection form used in IVF programs. Infertility itself does increase the risk of both these cancers, so that the best one could do to avoid the risk of them is to help the patient become pregnant. We do not know yet whether the extra eggs produced each month (in IVF cycles) would or would not bring on an early menopause; this will only be determined when studies are completed on couples as they pass the menopause. These studies are in progress.*

A patient comments: 'I had bowel problems and the doctor I saw said they were similar problems to a woman in her late forties or fifties taking HRT [hormone replacement therapy]. He said it had to do with the hormones. When I asked about the IVF drugs, he went quiet and re-stated his comparison with a woman on HRT.' Another adds:

You can't really criticise the doctors in regard to the drugs. All drugs have side-effects. Initially, it would be good to be made aware of the real side-effects of drugs, but then the doctors probably don't want you developing symptoms if you don't have them — just by suggestion. Everyone reacts differently. Some people I know have no problems at all with the drugs.

Chapter 16
Unconsummated Motherhood — Living without Children

'Children alone do not bring happiness and satisfaction in life.
Contentment isn't achieved through any one aspect of life.'

'I can describe childlessness. It's just like a tree, you have branches,
and you have branches that are the dead branches. I feel just like that, there
are no flowers on my branches.'

I have to be honest. I don't know how I would have felt if I hadn't had a child. I remember the bewilderment when I miscarried, asking myself what was wrong with me, why couldn't I do what other women did with such ease. I began investigations and treatment because I felt I wanted to try everything possible, and if that didn't work, I would at least have the comfort that I'd tried. I used to think that would sustain me, if a full-term pregnancy hadn't been possible.

I know my life would have been different. Within the chaos of leaving work, changing countries and caring for a toddler, I lost my creativity, the thing that had been my core all my life, and certainly during my twenty-five years of working on magazines. I found my total lack of external creativity frustrating, as did my husband, so used to me constantly working on a project of some kind.

I felt so lost and isolated, I went to see a psychologist. She listened intently to my story of life before and after my child and she smiled wisely and said: 'But of course, you've created the child you needed to have, the need to create other things has disappeared.'

There are losses and there are gains. My creative energy, if not absorbed by a child, may have gone on producing more magazines, or it may have changed course. The only certain thing is that whatever I did would have been single-minded, with no distractions.

Getting used to working during the school days has not been easy. My normal working pattern was full on, thinking of nothing else but magazines for twenty-four hours a day, seven days a week. It took me years after leaving work to stop choosing a magazine cover in my dreams or arranging the content, page by page. So the unconscious creativity remained, but the day-to-day dealing with the demands of a young child deadened that part of me just as it exposed other areas of tenderness that had previously been well armoured to deal with the rigours of a big, tough publishing company.

I feel very strongly that Daniel was not given exclusively to us. He has been called the 'village baby' since birth, and that is how I feel. He is not mine to possess totally as his mother — he has a select group of close people, some relatives, some friends, who form his family. Some haven't had their own children. Some have grown-up children. He is not a substitute child for anyone, but an extension of their lives. They enrich his life, he enriches theirs. He is an entity we are fortunate enough to parent, but he is himself.

How do those of us who were not successful resolve their loss? I know some who went through the experience and have truly worked through the pain. And also some who have simply buried the problem, never dealt with it, only to have it resurface intermittently with either bitterness or tears.

Someone close once said: 'You cannot imagine the bonds in a childless marriage. Bonds of guilt from the partner to *blame* and bonds of compassion from the other. So while the relationship may have its joy and light in other areas, on the issue of childlessness, there is a bond of shared sadness. And it's a very strong bond.'

Several women I know have made a definite choice not to have children. These are women who haven't simply come up with a barrage of pat reasons to keep people away from probing any pain.

Two of these women have been teachers, and they genuinely feel that their love and need for children has been amply satisfied in working with other people's children over many years. Another friend helped care for her sister's children, two of whom suffered from disabilities that required years of surgery and therapy. Although she tried at a later stage to have her own children and was unsuccessful, she now believes her feelings and emotional life have had the enrichment of children through these very close nephews. Others I know have been the eldest child in a family and helped raise the younger children. For them also, the maternal urge has been excised.

Maybe not everyone is suited to be a parent. The primeval urge to want children, however, is present in most of us, never more so than when we are told there is an impediment to our yearning. To hide our pain, we build up an impressive line of disinterest in the whole subject. Or we avoid it.

Family occasions, reunions, celebrations of Christmas or Mother's Day, christenings, all re-open the wound. I remember refusing to go to a high school reunion once. My parents thought I was being very unfriendly, ignoring my roots. I had another reason. I knew no matter how many magazines I'd produced, no matter what I'd achieved in my professional life, the two questions that would be asked of me by my *country cousins* would be: 'Are you married?' (no, not at the time, although my partnership was a longstanding one) and 'How many children do you have?'. It was this second question I couldn't face, so I avoided it.

No matter how much of me railed at being judged a success or not on whether I had married or reproduced, how unintelligent I thought the questions, the fact remained, I knew, in answer to the second question, I would be reduced to feeling a failure. No, I hadn't yet had any children. So I didn't go to the reunion and my former classmates thought I had become snobbish.

The national newsletter for ACCESS, Australia's national infertility network, published readers thoughts on how they get through their childless Christmas and Mother's Days. For Christmas, the most popular strategy was to get away somewhere and do something different, leaving a few days before Christmas and returning a few days afterwards — from a modest camping holiday by a river, to a more exotic trip to Bali. Then they share New Year holidays with family and friends, a time traditionally more adult in nature and therefore not quite so painfully linked with children and childlessness. Others chose to have a special meal at a Santa-free restaurant, or a quiet day at home together. More speak of their long Christmas morning in bed, perhaps envied by parents with shrieking children, quietly exchanging gifts, then a quiet lunch alone or bracing themselves for the full family assault, the latest pregnancy announced, the latest pram produced. Then returning to an empty house.

Mother's Day possesses a duality. At least one aspect is positive, in remembering and enjoying our mothers. However, the tender images in magazines and on television of mother and child intensify the grief for those who haven't had a longed-for child. And for those who have lost a child, either before birth or during infancy, the feelings are more poignant, as so many people forget that they have indeed had a taste of motherhood — one that was taken away.

Through my own experiences, I have learned never to ask the question 'do you have children?' I wait, I seek other ways to find out, because it can be the worst question of all if it comes at a vulnerable time. I remember a dinner where one friend who had two easily conceived children burbled on about the joys of motherhood. I looked at another (childless) friend across the table, knowing the discomfort she must have been feeling. Then, at some point, my childless friend made a general comment about children and my talkative friend blurted out that being a mother had given her such a wonderful new perspective on life that those without children could never understand. My childless friend exploded. Her nerves were too raw, perhaps the hour was too late. She said all the things she'd felt for years.

'Does this mean that those of us who haven't had children are less womanly, unable to feel. Are we second-class citizens, denied this superior wisdom?' she demanded. They were both devastated. The chatterbox because she hadn't wanted to hurt anyone, she was just filling in social spaces. My other friend because she saw it as a personal attack.

Most of us would agree that on a day we feel strong, comments such as this wouldn't be devastating. On a vulnerable day, however, they are like twisting a knife. How do you know when to stop if you've had years trying advanced reproductive technology? How do you decide to move on?

For someone close to me, it was giving away the knitting patterns: She said:

I've always loved to knit, so from the moment I became engaged I collected knitting patterns for baby clothes. I had a box of them and was so looking

Deirdre Bowie, in her book *Poems from the Heart* (Karibuni Press), describes her growing realisation of childlessness after many years of fertility treatment:

Spring Clean
I did a Spring Clean
Of our bookshelves recently.
I told the world
It was because we were moving house.
But I knew my children
Would never read
Would never need
These children's books
Bought over many years of anticipation
Looking forward to introducing
My children
To the world of Beatrix Potter,
To Pooh, Piglet and Eyeore,
To Peter Pan and Wendy
To Beauty and the Beast
To characters from my childhood
in Nursery Rhymes
Bible stories,
And Folk Tales
To the world of make-believe
Fantasy, magic and truth
The big books,
The small books,
The colourful and the drab

I packaged them lovingly that Spring —
Choosing these precious memories
For my young friends
These for Lizzie and Evie,
These for Adam and Petra
More favourites for Joshua and Zoe
And this pile for the Jones family
Heidi, Erica and Bonnie
My O-So-Special Nieces
Received the biggest pile of books
Gifts from a broken heart
Making tangible
The confirmation of our infertility.

Booklet available by writing to Deirdre Bowie, Karibuni Press, PO Box 81, Milperra NSW 2213, Australia.

forward to making things for our children. We were just in the days before IVF technology. I had to have surgery to investigate my fertility problems, a whole operation, not a laparoscopy like people have now. The diagnosis was endometriosis, with blocked tubes. So for us, pre-IVF, that was the end of it. Getting rid of the knitting patterns was the hardest thing to do in facing our infertility.

Some people re-channel their maternal instincts into their pets. Yet, for others, there is a fear and distaste over becoming maternal with a cat or a dog. One friend tells:

I have a very close girlfriend who married later in life to a much younger husband. When she tried to become pregnant and failed, she discovered she had had premature ovarian failure or early menopause. She explored the idea of donated eggs, but ultimately found she couldn't accept all the procedures and treatments that IVF with donor eggs would entail. She bought a cat. Now it is a very beautiful cat, but both she and her husband have become absolutely soppy about this animal. It has indeed become their substitute child. I look at them with faint horror and now I have found I can't conceive, I resist the idea of having an animal, knowing it may become a child-substitute for me too.

Others add:

I bought a budgie, it was the best thing I ever did.

I've got my dogs, they are my children.

I used to have my Siamese cat. He was the best companion imaginable. He sensed all my moods, *talked* as Siamese do and lay on my bed at times when I was trying to stay still to prevent an inevitable miscarriage. While I was pregnant with my son, I even dreamed I had given birth to a Siamese cat. When we arrived back in Australia with the new baby, we stayed with the friend who had adopted our cat in our absence. There was an amazing battle each time I fed the baby, seeing who could get closer to me, the cat or the baby.

For several years, my husband occasionally referred to our child by the cat's name. When the time to get a new cat arrived, several years after the Siamese had died, I found I wasn't as passionate about this cat as I had always been about others throughout my life. But whether that was because my child had filled the gap or whether it is just not a special cat, I'll never know. Another experience common to those who have failed to have children or those who had theirs with great difficulty is the pain they feel when they hear of an unwanted child, or abused or neglected children. People tell:

Coping so far with life without a child has been pure hell for me. My heart breaks every time I hear of an abused child, or one being left somewhere.

I had one girlfriend who had an abortion when I was going through infertility treatment. And I have never felt the same about her. It is not her fault, and I am not morally opposed to abortion, but I just couldn't deal with her aborting something I wanted so much.

Another woman explores her experiences with infertility, years of trying donor insemination, and finally giving up and coming to terms with her loss. She had treatment in what sounds like the Dark Ages, with possible ovulation indicated only by her own temperature taking. With only one insemination per month and no blood tests, by today's standards, it would seem a pretty haphazard treatment. Yet it was less than fifteen years ago. And she was being treated by the best specialist in her city. She tells her story of pain, hope and loss ... and rebuilding her life after giving up treatment:

There are certain days I remember vividly. Like the day I received the news that our closest friends were going to have a baby. She was about 42, always a hugely successful career person. I only heard later through mutual friends that she had always been broody. I remember the day I received her letter. Joe was taking me to work, I usually walked but it was raining. I collected my post on the way out and I said, 'Hey, there's a letter from Karen ... strange. Why is she writing to me?' We never wrote to each other, we just sent funny postcards if we were on holiday, and here was a long letter. I had to read it about four times and I said to Joe, 'You'll never believe this, Karen is pregnant.'

She had announced it in a jokey kind of way and it was a long, funny letter, about the changes she'd have to make to her wardrobe and who would have thought it would happen to her at her age. Obviously she'd been going through some major treatment for a long, long time, and she hadn't mentioned it. She was too close to just ring up and say, 'Guess what, I'm having a baby.'

I hadn't told her I was going through DI treatments. I always pretended I didn't want a baby, it only came out when her daughter was three or four. When she was born, we were there to see her first. It was a difficult one that. Because as infertile couples we've had this armour plate for so long, people think we are not vulnerable, we're always busy, far too busy to have children, that's certainly what we say.

This armour you put on, you convince even yourself, thinking I'm strong, I'm tough, I can handle this. Then suddenly you disintegrate — like with this letter. It happened more than once. While I was going through treatments thinking it's never going to happen, another close friend, who had two children already, arrived one night and said, 'You'll never guess what, I'm pregnant again.' There was something ridiculous like seventeen years between her other children. It really hurts, they come to visit and you have a lovely house and are having holidays and things like that, and they think you don't want children, but really you do.

Another day I remember vividly was the day I decided to stop treatments. I can tell you exactly when it happened, I can tell you the bit of pavement I was standing on. Carruthers was my gynaecologist. We called him 'Carruthers of the Foreign

Office'. He assured me they'd have me pregnant before the end of the year. We were working towards my 40th birthday — I'd been going there about two years. I went every month except during holidays or a major work project — basically nine months a year.

I went through all the stresses and strains common to most patients — trying to invent excuses to get away from the office for inseminations and appointments, driving round the block and fighting for a parking space. Then the 14-day wait — you think, please let it be food poisoning if you get a tummy ache, anything but your period, and that sinking feeling when it starts.

My temperature charts were never very steady, never classic. I had no hormone tests, I didn't know they existed. You put yourself totally in the doctors' hands and assume they will know everything and do everything.

Finally, I asked the doctor for guidance about treatments. He said, 'No it's OK, you've had all the tests, don't worry, it will happen.' Well it didn't.

After a while, it was around my 40th birthday, he said, 'I'm going to send you to see a colleague.' I asked why and he said he wanted another opinion. To find out a little more about me. This new doctor was silver-blonde haired, suave and elegant. He said, 'I don't know what you think about this because I can't see a problem, we can continue the treatments.' He said I had fibroids, but that didn't preclude a baby, but it just didn't seem to be happening. He added, 'We are quite prepared to carry on the treatment.' I said, 'What are the chances?'

'I can't tell you the chances, it's either going to happen or it's not,' he said. So I asked: 'What do you think?'

He said, 'There comes a time when you've got to think it's not going to happen.'

I didn't know any other options existed. I thought I was going to the top people, and this option was not working.

He told me not everyone wants children and I replied, 'Well, I do.'

He said other people want lots of boats and lots of houses and lots of clothes and lots of jewels, and I said I didn't want any of those things, I just wanted a baby. Now I see that some of this has come true — I seem to have lots of houses. What did he know? Suddenly I became very weak and tearful and I asked him did he have any children and he said he had two. I asked how he could know? He replied, 'I think for you it might be time to call it a day, but I am suggesting that to you, I'm not really telling you.'

I remember walking out feeling totally, totally empty, cold, nothing. And standing on the step feeling dead inside and dead in my brain. I asked myself where should I go from there. He had practically said to me that I was a no-go. I thought, *Why don't I do something else. Why don't I forget it, it's not going to happen.*

When I went to the local doctor (I'd had Clomid, then they gave me a prescription for something else) and I'd taken the new drug for a month they said take it to your doctor and get the prescription repeated. My doctor looked at me and he gave me a very strange look. He asked me, 'What is this for — why are you taking these? Who prescribed these?' I told him the gynaecologist he recommended I go to, 'Why?' He said, 'Because they're for cancer.' 'They're not,' I told him, 'they are for fertility.' He said, 'No, they are for cancer.' I said, 'I'm not taking them.' By that time my brain had switched off and I thought it's not going to happen and that's that. I was uncomfortable talking about it. I didn't to start with because it was terribly private and personal, you think you are exposing yourself, I found the whole thing, going to Carruthers and his gang anyway, seriously embarrassing, because I didn't have a rapport with them, they were perfectly nice, it was just impersonal.

My doctor kept saying I think I'll give up this business in a few years, I want to be an art dealer, so he'd want to talk to me about art instead. I said, 'I don't want to talk about that, that's not why I'm here.'

So standing on that pavement like cellophane man I decided that was that. The doctors never suggested any other kind of treatment like IVF with donor sperm, they suggested I continue what I was doing. But my head had had enough.

Two years is a long time, getting your period every month when you hope not to. I didn't start earlier because I was about 33 or 34 when we decided something was not working. In those days the woman was tested first. These tests took about a year and then we went to see someone about male testing. Joe had a nil count. We were never given a reason. The doctor was interested in doing research if he gave Joe an operation, but there seemed no point if he couldn't actually help us

We don't know what the problem was. Joe's parents came from big families. Something, an accident, happened to Joe when he was a child, something got into his penis. He had to have some sort of operation, then he was supposed to be OK. We were never given an actual reason he had no sperm.

I didn't start DI treatment then as I couldn't take it on board. I felt if we can't have a baby together, I won't have one at all. Joe asked how I felt about adoption, but that wasn't an option that I could entertain. I wanted to have my own in some way, it's not just looking after a child, for me, it has to have something of you in it. I know there are lots of children who need homes, but that wasn't the thing for me. It was Joe who kept suggesting DI and I kept saying no, then I thought if I don't try it, nothing is ever going to happen. So then it didn't work.

I was quite thin — I've always been a size 8 or a 10. I don't know whether it was subconscious — it obviously was, as no one likes gaining weight — but I suddenly found I was getting fat. I quite liked this, people thought I was pregnant. I used to wear big, blousey dresses like shifts and things — and people thought under there, there's a baby. It's all illusion. I was giving myself illusions.

The crunch came in Italy while we were on holiday, about two years after I stopped treatment. This was when I (subconsciously) thought I'll pretend I am pregnant. Overeating wasn't a conscious decision. I may have got to 11 stones, but I was perfectly happy with the situation. I went to work and everything was great. I was quite heavy. So on holiday, I went into the little local shop. My knowledge of the language wasn't great, but she obviously asked if I was pregnant and I automatically said 'Si.' Another part of me thought she had asked were we on holiday, or something like that. But I said YES to being pregnant. I suddenly realised what I'd said. And that shocked me to the core and I thought, *Wow, what a Freudian slip.*

I don't think I'd realised up till then what I was doing, like creating a phantom pregnancy. I wanted to feel what it was like to be fat, what it was like to have big boobs. The experience in the shop was like a detonator or the reverse of a detonator. Like turning a switch off. I didn't eat and I thought the time has come to face this, I was being stupid. I didn't know I was doing it. Finally, when I was below my normal weight, Joe said, 'Now stop it, you're getting like an Ethiopian chicken, your wrists are so thin, you're not eating anything.'

I wasn't trying to be anorexic, I was perfectly healthy about the whole thing. I just had a double reaction. I became sinewy, a total reverse to what I'd been subconsciously doing and I didn't even know I was doing it — till that woman in the shop in Italy. During this time, I was a voluptuous (read fertile) woman. A man at a dinner asked what did I like doing most? He said, 'I'm looking at you and you're eating, smoking, drinking.' I said I liked it all and that was that. At that stage I was overindulging in everything. I can't tell why, I didn't know what I was doing until that moment in the shop. I had a huge tummy.

Joe was supportive the whole way, soft and gentle. He would have loved to be a father as well. He backed whatever I wanted to do. When I announced I wasn't going back any more, he said fine, there was no question of pushing me to go and have any more treatments. He probably reckoned I'd had enough and my head had had enough. There comes a time when you have to give up.

We moved house and when new people came to live next door I remember thinking, she's having a baby, this is going to be hell, I'm not going to like her. We had moved to get away from all that and I'm going to have a baby next door to look at. But the child has turned out to be giving and loving, he could have been a thug. I was dreading the birth. Yet somehow, from the age he could walk this child chose me as his special alternative mother. I wanted to remain aloof, but he didn't allow it. He toddled around and appeared at the door. As soon as he could talk, he simply announced himself at the door with an 'It's me.' Now he has become one of the select group of children in my life. We have a special relationship quite different to the relationship he has with anyone else.

Have I resolved my childlessness? Maybe you never do, but I have moved on, into a new phase in my life. I have accepted it.

Now fertility treatment is more openly discussed, and I have read more, I sometimes wonder if I may have had a mental block to having a baby with donor sperm, that deep down I was worried that it may affect my relationship with Joe, and whether he would have coped. But that is now in the past.

Most women throw themselves into their careers more fully, take up higher education, use their energies in a different and positive way after they have given up treatment. The sex difference is important here, because men do not have to undergo the same often invasive treatments and hormone therapy that women do, even if the problem lies with the sperm. So the decision to give up is often a combination of physical, emotional and financial factors, but centring on the woman, who is the one being given treatment. So it is usually the woman who decides when she has had enough, in consultation with her partner. Doctors agree that the decision to stop or continue must be left to the patients. They can gently guide them to the decision, but ultimately they cannot make it.

Some women, like Sandra Dill, the Executive Director of ACCESS, Australia's national infertility network, have combined further education with stimulating jobs. She formed ACCESS, helping others who are undergoing infertility treatment.

IVF Friends Inc., Melbourne, published a letter in their bulletin, in which a reader asked: 'Is there anyone out there who has made their life complete without children?'

One of the replies was later published in their book *IVF Letters: Personal Experiences of IVF*, published by IVF Friends Inc., Melbourne, Australia. In it, the reader listed her failed treatments and the physical aspects of these, familiar to many.

She told how she stopped treatments at the time her very dominant father became ill and eventually died. Her grief for her father and her childlessness compounded, and she said she became so low that there was no place else to go but up.

She began to talk with her mother and to learn from her mother's attempts to overcome her grief. Her mother told her she had settled on two resolutions: that life is what you make of it and to make sure she didn't glorify her husband, choosing to remember the bad things along with the good. Her mother said at one point that she had decided life wasn't complete without a partner, so she told her daughter she was lucky to have her husband. The daughter said you are lucky to have me, asking 'Who has everything?'

This reader then began to look at the negatives of children as well as the more romanticised image of shining faces and hair, and angelic smiles at bedtime. She suddenly started to look at the harried faces of women in supermarkets dealing with tired children throwing tantrums, the financial sacrifices her friends were making. Basically, she explored the down-side of parenting, too. She said she realised children alone couldn't bring happiness. They couldn't mend a marriage or fix a failing career. She acknowledged, as many other women have throughout interviews for this book, that the powerful drive to have a child and the ensuing treatments, blot out other aspects of your life that may not be working.

Other women have acknowledged that even if they do end up with a THB ('take-home baby'), they still have to get back to normal life and deal with normal things, such as the state of their relationships or the disrepair in their houses. Although they often feel if they end up with a child, they'll never ask for another thing in life, human nature isn't like that. As soon as we get something we badly want, its importance diminishes and the other problems and wants resurface.

The Melbourne woman concluded that life is made up of a variety of aspects or boxes. Children are one of these aspects, but marriage, career, relationships with friends and family, and lifestyle were other aspects. So if she wasn't able to have children, she would utilise the energies she had allocated for children making other aspects of her life better, for both her and her husband. She said that five years after giving up treatment, she could finally say she was happy, but that during those five years she had had to go on a long and powerful emotional journey.

Chapter 17
Helping Ourselves, Helping Others

The Role of Support Groups in Infertility Management

'It's like a lifeline, You need to laugh, as long as you are laughing
with it, not at it. People in the same position can do that.'

~e~

'Australia has benefited greatly from fertility support groups.'
**Dr Stephen Steigrad, Director of Reproductive Medicine,
Royal Hospital for Women, Randwick, NSW, Australia**

Infertility is an isolated and isolating experience.

Joining a support group can help modify some of these feelings of being alone, and provide you with a nourishing supply of new friends who share and understand the complex experiences. Support groups can also supply you with fact sheets on the very latest treatments, give you information about the various clinics and specialists, and also provide you with up-to-date information on legislation covering assisted reproductive technology. In most countries, there are one or two major groups, which usually have a central registry of affiliated groups around the country so that they can suggest one close to where you live.

Many couples don't tell anyone of their quest for a child. It therefore comes as a great relief after joining a support group to find that they are not alone in the emotions they are facing. The experiences are universal, with minor variations depending on your particular medical scenario.

While most clinics do provide counsellors (in Australia they are obligatory), many patients find they can unload more of their feelings with each other than with a counsellor. They think that if they expose their difficulty in coping to a counsellor, it may be prejudicial to their case for continuing treatment. Counsellors are also medical professionals, and many people still feel intimidated when dealing with the medical profession and don't expose their inner struggles to them. Many clinics display leaflets about fertility support groups. If they don't, the best idea is to telephone the national network in your country and they will give you information about the group dealing with your specific treatment in your area.

A woman from Queensland, Australia, talks about the beginnings of her involvement with a group:

I found a support group newsletter and left it on the table for my husband to read and initially he came to meetings reluctantly, but gradually he got involved. We had just moved here and didn't have many friends. I worked for a Japanese company and he is in the police force, so we didn't really want to share our problems with our work associates. So the support group also became a good social outlet for us. It takes males longer to accept infertility, my husband just didn't want to get outside help. I felt I really needed someone to talk to.

Her husband said:

In the newsletter it said just come along, you won't get a job. Five minutes after arriving, I found I was president of the group. It's the best thing we ever did. People are so secretive, I think that's a problem. They think it is better keeping it that way, but you are much better in a group talking about it, at least you can laugh about it.

To which the wife added:

If you want to be down in the mouth and depressed, people in the group don't just pat you on the back and say 'There, there' like your mother or a friend. They will talk to you, ask you which cycle you are on, you can relate to them. And if you want to crack a funny, you can, like saying 'Do you know what happened to me as I was lying with my legs up in the air ...' — you can laugh about it. If you were at a barbecue with a normal group of friends and you bring it up, they suddenly all turn away or disappear into the kitchen and you're left there alone, thinking. People don't want to know or be involved with it. Here we just laugh and laugh, and it's healthy. I've never had to buy so many clothes since I joined our group.

Because parents using donor sperm and eggs often face unique dilemmas, they have their own support group, as do those suffering frequent miscarriages. Some patients with specific health problems such as endometriosis have also created their own groups. The national networks — ACCESS in Australia, ISSUE or CHILD in the United Kingdom, RESOLVE in the United States and The New Zealand Infertility Society Inc. — can all give the information you require.

There is also a group called the International Federation of Infertility Patient Associations (IFIPA) which unites sixteen national associations from twelve countries. This group's mission is to join the world's infertility patient associations and so increase global awareness and challenge cultural taboos surrounding infertility.

These support groups provide much more than a social network of caring friends. They act as consumer advocates for the rights of the infertile in the formation of laws and government policies, they publish newsletters which bring patients up-to-the-minute information from the medical profession. They also print specific leaflets on myriad subjects connected with infertility and, because these are leaflets rather than books, they are updated frequently so you are likely to find the latest methods of treatment from the top doctors in each field.

The national networks can also give information about clinics in your area and usually have a helpline, a list of sympathetic fellow-patients people can call for advice or moral support.

In Australia, ACCESS was born at the end of its founder's battle with infertility.

Sandra Dill AM, appointed to the Order of Australia in the Queen's Birthday Honours List in 1996 for her services as a consumer advocate in the area of infertility, is the executive director and founder of ACCESS. She is quick to stress that her work came from a need to create something positive from her twelve years of unsuccessful treatment for unexplained or idiopathic infertility.

It is, however, the most inspiring story of how someone dealing with pain and depression after years of unsuccessful treatment became an advocate with doctors and government to get a better deal for patients of the future.

SANDRA DILL'S STORY

ACCESS was formed out of an old association, the National Fertility Association, which was about to fold. I have a background in management, so I put together a business proposal and walked it around a lot of people. I just didn't want to see us lose the gains we had made in recognition of infertility as a serious medical problem, particularly with the medical profession. We had representation on their accredited body, which was unique in Australia at the time and may still be, and we had representation on their federal council. Establishing credibility there took a lot of years to achieve, and I didn't want to lose it all. I think that my motivation to do all this was for a few different reasons, but it primarily grew from my own experience of infertility.

For me, one way of dealing with it or coping was to do something constructive. In a sense, that's a very selfish motivation because I needed to get involved. It wasn't altruistic at all. Some people cope by disappearing, I just wanted to have some control. I was also interested in politics, therefore I was interested in the access consumers had to the technology and to safety issues, so my interest drew me to a continuing involvement after I stopped treatment.

My experience of infertility began this involvement. My treatment days spanned out over about fourteen years. I have idiopathic [unexplained] infertility. I went to my gynaecologist when I didn't become pregnant normally and, after five years of work-up tests, I was referred for IVF. I was on a three-year waiting list in those days, but got to the top within two and a half years. My husband and I went to Professor Saunders at Sydney's Royal North Shore Hospital. I took a list of twenty-nine questions, much to my husband's embarrassment. He sat looking at the door wondering when he could leave. I thought I was really well informed, I knew what my chances were. They were less than 10 per cent of taking home a baby. The THB [take-home baby] rate we call it!

On my first day of treatment, I was introduced to Judy. I don't know who she was, I've never seen her since. And they suggested that Judy might take me to where the scans were being done. And it occurred to me that she'd obviously been through this before as she knew where the scanner was. As we walked out the door I said, 'You've been here before' and she told me this was her fourth attempt.

I felt like someone had kicked me in the stomach — but what a curious response, given that I knew my chances were low. I learned then and later had it reinforced many times: your intellectual response is one thing, but your emotional response is an entirely different thing. And particularly when there is nothing wrong with you and there's never been anything wrong with you. You think there is some glitch there. My greatest fear in my first cycle was that I'd have quads. Which I'm amused at now. Even with triplets — naturally conceived triplets as well — 70 per cent of couples are divorced within five years. That's why at ACCESS we keep pushing the idea that multiple births are not a good outcome.

When it didn't work the first time that was very disappointing. We went back again, because we had good attempts, we got eggs and they fertilised with my husband's sperm. On our fourth attempt, we did achieve a pregnancy. And that was amazing … and I miscarried at 14 weeks. My mother had been asking what kind of cot I wanted, she was so delighted after our nine years of trying. I said to leave it a little bit longer. Someone said after 12 weeks I should be confident now. I told Mum, 'No, just wait a bit longer.'

And at 14 weeks, my husband called her at 1.30 in the morning to say we were at the hospital and I had miscarried.

Looking back, I have different responses to that. I wish I'd never been pregnant. It raises your hopes and, though you're very guarded, you allow yourself to feel joy that you've finally achieved the dream of becoming a parent. So all that seemed quite cruel, but I thought that's life. I had one lady say to me at least I knew I could be pregnant. I said I'll tell you what it was like to lose my child, I'll give you a minute-by-minute description of what it felt like to have my baby pulled out of me in pieces and seeing it put in this pristine white stainless steel dish in this seriously pristine white linen towel. It was all very orderly, but it is something I'll never forget. There was no joy at all for me in knowing that I was pregnant, pregnancy wasn't the goal, it was having the baby at the end of the time.

We kept going for another four attempts. My very final attempt was a frozen cycle. I had three frozen embryos. The three clinic sisters were away sick and the poor scientist had the job of ringing all the women and telling them if their embryos had survived the thaw. Scientists are very clinical, they don't like talking. If they have to, they talk about the viability of the embryo — and I asked are they dead or alive. I could hear him gulp. He said they are viable, but you can't tell till they are properly thawed. He said he couldn't keep looking as they were in a controlled environment. I said 'OK, I'm not coming in to be told they are dead.'

I was deliberately using language that would shock him. I wasn't trying to be difficult, these were my potential children, I didn't want to talk about them being viable or non-viable — they were my children. The poor guy, I rang him about four times and, when they had completed the thaw process, he gave me the news that only one had survived.

I told him it was hardly worth coming in, because I knew what the chances were and I didn't want to have to go through that dreadful two-week wait. I was at my brother's place at Neutral Bay. One of the nurses called and told me I was supposed to be in there (it was only ten minutes away). I told her I just didn't see the point. She was really good and I could hear the doctor in the background saying 'Sandra, get your arse in here.'

She finally said, 'OK, you make the decision, but if you decide to do it you need to be here within half an hour.'

I sat down and thought for about five minutes and realised I couldn't just leave that embryo there and I went in and they had a registrar on and I just loathe ebullient registrars and he was an identical twin of a journalist I know, so it was a bit unnerving. He told me he'd done two single embryo transplants in the last month and both had gone on to achieve a pregnancy. 'Well brace yourself,' I said, 'I'm probably about to break your run.'

It didn't work, but it was not altogether a surprise. I was then 39 and I wanted to have another go and my husband said twelve of the fourteen years of our marriage we'd been trying to get pregnant, and was that what our lives had become. Which was a pretty reasonable question.

That was a very difficult time. I recognised that it was a reasonable question, but I felt like the control about whether or not I'd have a child had been taken from me. I wanted to make the decision. Now we both feel we would have handled it differently — I was just very driven. In conversations later, he said I would never have stopped. I probably would have kept going until I was about 42 because I realistically knew it wouldn't happen after then. But my husband explained that we were just going into debt and we weren't doing anything else. You need to put your life on hold to some extent because the treatment is so intrusive.

Throughout that we were involved in the local support group.

After I stopped, I was depressed for about eighteen months. I had counselling and they told me that what I was suffering was acute reactive depression and grief. I didn't have any drugs or anything, I just talked to people. There was a profound sense of alienation and I was confronted with was the final removal of all hope that I'd ever be a parent. And that was extraordinarily difficult to come to terms with.

I recall about two months after this initially happened, I kept on going to work and doing the things I was doing, and I was speaking at a seminar for a support group thinking what on earth could I say that was positive. The thing about that was I was forced to try and think of something good and the things that occurred to me were that I was grateful about being able to make a choice through IVF and that was an option not available twenty years before that. And the hurt that flowed from not achieving a baby was not a lot different to the hurt that appears at other times throughout our lives.

I've done some interviews since then and people have said to me IVF should be banned as it's too painful and women shouldn't have to go through that — and

I've thought about it and I now say that we all make choices about things we'd like to pursue in our lives. And most of our decisions come at a cost — we pursue them because we believe the goals we have chosen to pursue are worthwhile. Our choice, as patients using advanced reproductive technology, is to try to have a child. Saying you shouldn't do something because it causes you pain is pointless — we all do things that are difficult or for which there is a cost involved.

You can always look back as a couple and say we gave it our best shot. I guess I need to believe sometimes you attempt things because they are important to you and not necessarily because they are possible. If you didn't get the outcome you wanted, at least you did endeavour to do it.

During my treatment, I was asked to appear on a television program about IVF on the ABC, documenting a whole cycle. The visibility I found difficult, it was like reliving the failed attempt in front of a million people. But afterwards women would come to me and ask: 'What are we going to do as childless people, we don't fit in any more, we can't really relate to people who have children, we don't even have the same interests. It is not just the emotional aspect of having no children, we just don't have the same interests. What are we going to do?'

I was very relieved others had those problems, I was beginning to feel there was something wrong with me. That is what motivated me to form ACCESS.

I had people coming to me telling me how altruistic I was, arguing for Medicare rebates and similar things. But I think in doing this it was really motivated by my child-lessness. I don't have a child and I can't now have a child because of my age. I am an infertile person, I am a childless person, and I will live with the impact of that forever.

What I have learned to do in painfully small, incremental steps is to learn how to manage what comes with that. You make specific choices. Once you've been depressed, you don't want to go back and live with that again because its pretty scary. What you learn, what you are forced to face is: Do I want to be happy? What do I want from life? Certainly this has been devastating, but for how long am I going to let this bury me?

I think in the end what I wanted was something really small — to find joy in everyday things again. That seemed to me to be really important. And to be able to find other goals and pursue them. I went back to university. It took me a few semesters to get into it, my fear of failure was still around. That fear of failure was quite dramatic. After the first semester, I completed all other aspects of my course, but I withdrew just before the exams because I couldn't step up to that line — and I couldn't cope with any more disappointment. I fought my way back gradually doing more, taking one subject not three to begin with. And slowly you begin to move on.

Other women sometimes ask for advice and I say I have learned a great deal about not giving advice to anyone. But if I had to do one thing differently, I would try to run some other interest concurrently, something that didn't take up a lot of time, because logistically treatment takes up a lot of time. I think you need something else that means something to you, otherwise if you end up with disappointment, then you have nothing.

I will only say to women to find something else that is important — something small—to put steps in place for the future. Because I really hope it works for them, but for many it doesn't. I wish I had done this—I was so disappointed at the time, I didn't have a lot of energy to set something up.

In some respects ACCESS became that. After taking my proposal around many organisations, it was finally launched in 1993. It was great, we got coverage on all the TV channels so that was really exciting. Doctors have given their financial support, saying the level of information we give their patients is so good that it helps them.

What gained me a lot of support in Australia was that when we were negotiating Medicare rebates for treatments, the question of accreditation and accountability of fertility clinics came up. I felt that if clinics have the privilege of coverage under the national public health system, public accountability must arise, and we had no accreditation body. The medical profession said they were a self-regulating body and were working on an accreditation system.

Very soon after this came a situation in Perth where a clinic and its head doctor were found to be acting irresponsibly and accreditation was withheld. The government body was thrilled when we went to the next meeting, knowing we were really serious about this. The doctors found it worked in their favour. They could say: 'Look here we have a consumer on the committee. No one can say we are gynaecologists and talk in a patronising manner to non-medical people. We have a consumer on our accreditation panel and she sees everything; we are willing to be completely open.' The lateral thinkers among the medical profession saw this would be a good strategy. So every time they speak on anything controversial, they can repeat this. And it deflects public distrust. It is a good strategy on their part.

Support groups around Australia are linked to ACCESS, but not in a legal way. We have a central group register nationally—so if people contact us we send them the ACCESS information and put them in touch with a group near where they live. We also contact these groups for feedback if anything unusual happens. If I go to a meeting, this ensures what I discuss is representational.

Sometimes male partners don't like the idea of talking about going to a support group. I know when once we said we were going to have a discussion group meeting, the men felt they could come. I would always encourage people to speak with someone else who has been through a similar experience because they will find it makes the whole experience a little less isolating for them.

Most people who have been through the infertility experience agree the one question you never ask others is whether they have children. I used to feel very defensive about the question. What I say now when people ask me is 'No.' Just very quietly, then I move on with the conversation. I don't feel the need to explain. I try to move the conversation on so they don't have the opportunity to pursue the topic and I've really never had anyone come back and ask me further. I think it's in the way you say no.

It usually happens in the first five minutes of a conversation, so I don't just sit there and leave a silence. And I never ask people do they have children now. If I pick up that they do I might ask how they are. I used to feel I had to explain that I was trying. Now I don't think I have any obligation to tell people whether I have children.

I don't have to explain why I don't have them either. If someone were to ask me directly why I don't have any — depending on how mischievous I was feeling — I'd like to say something to shock them.

If I thought it was intrusive, I tell them it was a very personal question. Before I used to feel I had to take care of people, so they didn't feel uncomfortable. Now I might say I suffer from infertility. It kills the conversation pretty quickly. At a cocktail party once I was going to go into details about my husband and I having difficulty, but I was really tired. I was trying to say it softly then I thought, what the heck, so I said I was infertile — it was like a bomb had gone off. I thought great, I don't have to say any more. People feel they don't quite know what to say. It just confirms the idea this is something we are very uncomfortable with, still.

In my university class of about nine people, all younger than me, after a presentation I gave on anti-discrimination law, the others asked me what I did. When I told them I was a consumer advocate for infertile people, a young guy of about 18 started saying Westmead Hospital needs sperm donors and he thought he'd go along and give it a go. I asked how he knew he would be accepted. He replied that of course he would.

'Do you have any children?' I asked. 'You don't know that you can, do you?' There was stunned silence and the lecturer smiled and then we chatted a bit and the young guy asked how could I talk about this. I thought, I bet you tell all the dirty jokes under the sun. I explained that for the people going through infertility, it is a really serious business so talking about the *wanking room* — or something else they thought was cute — was really serious. For an infertile couple, when a woman is in theatre after undergoing hormone injections for a couple of weeks and she's lying there unconscious with doctors there waiting, if you are the husband and you have to deliver that semen sample, there's nothing amusing about it, there's too much riding on it.

'Well, when you put it like that ...' he said. We got into a conversation about why everyone was so nervous talking about infertility and the lecturer came up with an interesting perspective. He said when you talk about our ability not to have children you're striking at the very core of our identity, of who we are. And the idea that someone might suggest to us that we might not be able to have a child at the time we choose suddenly raises a whole lot of issues about whether there will be people coming after us — this is an assumption that if you grow up and become an adult you can have a child. And initially the concern is more that you don't have an unwanted pregnancy.

So when you talk about infertility, it's almost like people think if they talk to you about it they are interested and if they are interested maybe they have a problem. And no one wants anyone to think that. It has nothing to do with a man's virility, but that's the perception that is there. It needs to be opened up and looked at. It's another medical problem, but it's a very emotional one.

It would be good if we could come to it with a little less mysticism surrounding it. And the more open discussion we can generate on the subject, the more likely that is to be. And ACCESS plans to continue that discussion.

Doctors around the world recognise the importance of national support bodies for infertile couples. As Dr Stephen Steigrad says:

Australia has benefited from fertility support groups, now linked through a national consumer group called ACCESS. They were instrumental in making sure there was Medicare rebate for treatment. Several years ago there was a move in the federal Labor Party to exclude fertility treatment and there was a huge nationwide lobby where we pushed the politicians. The national fertility awareness body got really stuck into them and made them backpedal like fury because they knew they would have lost votes. The result was we got rebates for treatments. However, Brian Howe, the then Minister for Health, put a limit of six IVF treatments on it. There is absolutely no reason for that, except that I'm told he said that no woman would want to go through it more than six times. Six times in a woman's lifetime. Which means there is no room to try for a second child.

All over the world, each time cost cutting is discussed within a national health scheme, infertility treatment is spotlighted, as though it is a luxury. Sandra Dill's loss in her fight to have a family is the gain of infertile couples throughout Australia as she uses her energy and considerable persuasive powers to fight at all levels on behalf of fellow sufferers.

Interestingly, the formation of the two main national groups in the United Kingdom was also carried out by people who were patients.

CHILD was founded by a woman called Dorothy Bull, an infertility patient who felt there was no group solely for people with infertility — other groups included The Voluntarily Childless. It was founded in 1979 and formed into a trust, and originally run on a voluntary basis, with the support of two fertility specialists, Peter Niven and Robert Winston. Like ACCESS, it produces a newsletter packed with information, personal stories, the latest breakthroughs, names to ring on the Support Helpline. It also has a comprehensive series of fact sheets, dealing individually with problems contributing to infertility.

ISSUE, the other major group in the United Kingdom, does similar work, and both band together to promote Infertility Awareness Week each year, in the hope that as the public become better informed about the issues of infertility, they will become more understanding of the distress caused by infertility. ISSUE was founded in 1976 when Peter Houghton wrote a letter to a national newspaper about the emotions experienced during infertility and asking if anyone in that situation would be interested to meet others. There were more than 400 letters in response. Later, a meeting was held in Birmingham, and the National Association for the Childless was formed, which later became ISSUE (the National Fertility Association).

RESOLVE, the umbrella group for infertility support groups in the USA, is similar to other national bodies, publishing a newsletter, offering information sheets on all infertility-related topics, and serving as an advocate for issues such as legislation and insurance. It offers support groups, counselling, physician referrals and telephone helplines and provides information on clinics and treatments. RESOLVE was founded in 1974 as a non-profit organisation by Barbara Eck Menning, with the aim to produce 'timely, compassionate support and to increase awareness of infertility issues through public education and advocacy'.

The New Zealand Infertility Society Incorporated was founded in 1990 to provide support for a national network for infertile people; a national voice on infertility issues; advocacy to improve access to effective, equitable publicly funded services; links between the infertile and infertility specialists; information about all aspects of infertility; raised awareness in the community; representation on medical, legal, ethical and policy issues; to ensure people make informed life-choices to protect their fertility, and to establish a fund for postgraduate research into all aspects of infertility. It is also affiliated with ACCESS in Australia and is a member of the international body IFIPA.

Through groups like these, no one need ever suffer alone. As one patient said, receiving the response from her letter to a local support group was like receiving 'a hug in an envelope'. During infertility, we need all the hugs we can get.

Useful Addresses

ACCESS
Australia's National Infertility Network
PO Box 959
Parramatta NSW 2124
Australia

CHILD
Charter House
43 St Leonard's Road
Bexhill-on-Sea, East Sussex TN40 1JA
United Kingdom

COTS
Childlessness Overcome through
Surrogacy
Loandhu Cottage
Gruids, Lairg
Sutherland IV27 4EF
Scotland
United Kingdom

DI Network
PO Box 265
Sheffield S3 7YX
United Kingdom

Donor Conception Support Group
PO Box 53
Georges Hall NSW 2198
Australia

ISSUE
The National Fertility Association
114 Lichfield Street
Walsall
West Midlands WS1 1SZ
United Kingdom

New Zealand Infertility Society Inc.
PO Box 34 151
Birkenhead
Auckland 1330
New Zealand

RESOLVE
1310 Broadway
Somerville
Maryland 02144–1731
United States of America

Leonie McMahon
23 Beaumont Street
Killara NSW 2071
Australia

Paul Entwistle
The Rodney Fertility Clinic
37 Rodney Street
Liverpool L1 9EN
United Kingdom

Index